Hèla Ben Jmaà
Faten Dhouib
Rania Hammami

Surgical revascularization of lesions of the left common trunk

Surgical revascularization of lesions of the left common trunk

Hèla Ben Jmaà
Faten Dhouib
Rania Hammami

Surgical revascularization of lesions of the left common trunk

Atheromatous lesions of the left common trunk

ScienciaScripts

Imprint

Any brand names and product names mentioned in this book are subject to trademark, brand or patent protection and are trademarks or registered trademarks of their respective holders. The use of brand names, product names, common names, trade names, product descriptions etc. even without a particular marking in this work is in no way to be construed to mean that such names may be regarded as unrestricted in respect of trademark and brand protection legislation and could thus be used by anyone.

Cover image: www.ingimage.com

This book is a translation from the original published under ISBN 978-620-6-71602-0.

Publisher:
Sciencia Scripts
is a trademark of
Dodo Books Indian Ocean Ltd. and OmniScriptum S.R.L publishing group

120 High Road, East Finchley, London, N2 9ED, United Kingdom
Str. Armeneasca 28/1, office 1, Chisinau MD-2012, Republic of Moldova, Europe
Printed at: see last page
ISBN: 978-620-3-22131-2

Surgical revascularisation of atheromatous lesions of the left common trunk

I. Introduction:

A significant lesion of the left coronary common trunk (LCCT) is greater than or equal to 50% of the reference diameter. It is found in 5 to 7% of pathological coronary angiograms, and is often associated with multi-truncular involvement. (1).

The aims of myocardial revascularisation in patients with tight CKGR stenosis are to treat angina, improve left ventricular function, prevent myocardial infarction and improve the quality of life and life expectancy of coronary patients.

From the very beginning of the history of trans-cutaneous angioplasty, TCCG was a target, with initial disappointing attempts by Hartzler (2).

In addition, the CASS study confirmed the indisputable benefit of coronary artery bypass graft (CABG) surgery compared with medical treatment in terms of survival in patients with CKGR stenosis. Surgical treatment then became the reference treatment for these lesions (3).

The progress made in interventional cardiology since the advent of active stents, the emergence of safe anti-platelet agents, and the growing experience of operators, have led us to take up the challenge of percutaneous revascularisation of unprotected TCCG with greater ease and safety.

However, stenoses of the TCCG are rarely isolated and are often associated with multi-truncular involvement; they are often distal and involve bifurcations, areas at high risk of restenosis and thrombosis, and they are calcified in almost half of cases.

These anatomical features and the complexity of the lesions represent major technical limitations for angioplasty, whereas they are easily bypassed by an arterial or venous graft during surgical revascularisation.

The respective roles of these two techniques are the subject of controversy, and the publication of the SYNTAX study has fundamentally reopened the debate. (3). Several other randomised trials have shown that angioplasty with active stents offers long-term survival rates comparable to those with surgical revascularisation using coronary bypass grafts (4).

The choice of treatment and the myocardial revascularisation strategy depend on the patient's clinical profile and the angiographic characteristics of the coronary lesions.

However, elements of consensus are beginning to emerge, such as the need for a multi-disciplinary approach with the concept of the "Heart team", a repositioning of the patient at the centre of a debate in which his opinion and choices remain essential, and finally the use of scores combining clinical and angiographic data to guide the revascularisation strategy (SYNTAX score, SYNTAX clinical score and SYNTAX score II).

II. Definition and incidence of stenosis of the left coronary common trunk :

Significant stenosis of the TCCG is defined as a reduction of 50% or more in the diameter of the arterial lumen (5) (6).

The prevalence of tight stenosis of the TCCG is 5 to 10% of coronary angiographies performed for suspected or known coronary disease. (7) (8) (9). The frequency of isolated involvement of the TCCG varies from less than 0.5% to 1% of patients having undergone coronary angiography according to the different series (10) (11).

III.   Clinical profile of patients with left common stenosis :

1- Age :

In a recent study published by Zheng et al (7)the average age of patients operated on was 62.2 +/- 9.1 years. These data are consistent with those found in the literature (9) (12) (13).

2- Gender:

Male predominance has been reported in several studies, with the proportion ranging from 73% to 94%. (14) (15) (16) (17) (9).

Topaz et al (11) in a series of 21545 patients who underwent coronary angiography, identified 16 patients with stenosis of the TCCG without associated lesions on the main coronary trunks, with an equal distribution between the two sexes (50% men and 50% women).

3- Cardiovascular risk factors :

Cardiovascular risk factors in patients with CKGR stenosis are not specific. In fact, their incidence and distribution are no different from those found in other coronary diseases. Only familial hypercholesterolaemia is more specifically associated with stenosis of the common trunk of the left coronary artery (18).

The C.A.S.S study (Coronary Artery Surgery Study), which included 24958 patients, 1484 of whom had a tight stenosis of the TCCG, showed a classic predominance of smoking (frequency 76%), hypertension 38%, diabetes 16% and dyslipidaemia 45%. (19).

The rate of diabetics was 28% in the SYNTAX (20) and 32% in the PRECOMBAT (21).

In another study conducted by Boudriot between 2003 and 2009, which included 201 patients with significant stenosis of the TCCG, hypertension came first with a frequency of 82%, followed by dyslipidaemia (66.5%), then diabetes (36.5%). Smoking comes fourth with a frequency of 31.5%. (22).

In another study conducted by CHENG CI between 2000 and 2007, which included 363 patients with significant stenosis of the TCCG, smoking ranked fourth with a frequency of 26.4%, after hypertension (70.4%), dyslipidaemia (59.4%) and diabetes (45.3%) (23).

As in the case of other coronary diseases, the accumulation of risk factors increases the probability of CGRT disease and the likelihood of associated coronary lesions.

Indeed, in his series including patients with isolated stenosis of the TCCG, Revault (24) reported an average of 1.45 risk factors per patient.

4. History of coronary heart disease :

The notion of a history of previous coronary disease in relation to the diagnosis of CKGR stenosis has been found in several studies (22) (23) (25).

Cavalcante et al (26)in a recent study published in 2016, noted a history of coronary disease in 16.7% of patients undergoing TCCG surgery, 6.3% of whom had undergone stenting.

In the C.A.S.S study, which included 1484 patients with a lesion of the TCCG, 45% had a history of myocardial infarction (19).

5. Other atheromatous sites:

Cavalcante et al (26) noted the presence of a history of peripheral vascular disease in 7.1% of the population studied and a history of stroke in 4.1%.

6. Chronic renal failure :

In the series by Cavalcante et al (26)the mean creatinine clearance was 81+/-27.7 ml/min.

7. Clinical presentation :

The clinical presentation of CKGR stenosis can vary from completely asymptomatic to sudden death (27).

1. Acute coronary syndrome, myocardial infarction and stress angina :

Seung et al (28) showed in a recent study including 2238 patients with significant stenosis of the TCCG that the clinical presentation is dominated by acute coronary syndrome (ACS) (57.6%), followed by stable exertional angina (26%) and non-Q-wave myocardial infarction (10.9%).

The myocardial infarction revealing the lesion of the TCCG is generally related to an occlusion of a collateral coronary artery other than the TCCG.

Several studies have demonstrated the rarity of this clinical presentation of CGRT stenosis: in the study by Boudriot (22)only 13% of patients had a myocardial infarction. Lee Young (29) showed a lower rate of myocardial infarction at 3.9%.

The GRACE registry (Global Registry of Acute Coronary Events), whose database included 43,000 patients, among whom 1,799 cases of ACS with significant stenosis of the TCCG could be identified, showed that ACS with stenosis of the TCCG is a rare and severe situation. In fact, this situation was noted in only 4% of patients (30).

Table I summarises the various studies:

Table I: Clinical presentation according to studies.

Studies	Number of patients	Clinical presentation = MI (%)
Boudriot (22)	201	13
Lee Young (29)	509	3,9

| Park (21) | 223 | 8 |
| Seung (31) | 2340 | 10,2 |

2. Silent ischaemia :

The frequency of asymptomatic truncal stenosis varies in the literature. In the CASS (19)study, only 3.6% of patients with significant stenosis of the TCCG were symptomatic (14).

Seung (28) in his recent series of 2240 patients, reported a frequency of asymptomatic forms of 2.7%.

3. Dyspnoea :

Dyspnoea is associated with diffuse ischaemia and left ventricular dysfunction. This symptom does not appear to be more frequent than in other coronary diseases.

Carrie (32)in a study of 134 patients, reported dyspnoea as the clinical presentation of CKGR stenosis in only 7% of cases, 4% of whom had acute lung oedema.

8. Clinical examination :

The physical examination is often without abnormalities. It may also reveal signs of repercussions of stenosis of the trunk on cardiac function, such as signs of left heart failure or even pulmonary oedema, or anomalies related to valvular or vascular damage associated with coronary damage.

IV- Additional tests:

1. Resting electrocardiogram (ECG) data :

Resting ECG is not predictive of common trunk stenosis and has no localising value (33).

It is most often abnormal, revealing signs of ischaemia and/or sequelae of myocardial infarction. On the other hand, a normal ECG can be seen in 20% of cases and cannot exclude a pathology of the trunk, which is in favour of the poor sensitivity of this test. (32).

Changes in the ST segment in AVR when the TCCG is involved have also been described by Yamaji (34)who analysed the ECGs of 16 patients with obstruction of the TCCG, 46 patients with obstruction of the ostial segment of the IVA and 24 patients with obstruction of the right coronary artery.

This author concluded that AVR elevation of more than 0.5 mm was significantly more frequent in the course of MCCT damage than in the other coronary segments.

Another very evocative electrical aspect was described by Sclarovsky's team (35). It consists of a circumferential pattern of subendocardial lesions and subepicardial ischaemia explained by the fact that occlusion or severe stenosis of the TCCG leads to an acute increase in LV end-diastolic pressure without any increase in LV blood volume.

2. Stress ECG data :

Exercise stress testing is the most widely used non-invasive diagnostic method for detecting myocardial ischaemia. This test can detect myocardial damage, estimate the extent of ischaemia, assess the functional value of the myocardium and evaluate the prognosis. (36).

The stress ECG is most often positive in cases of significant lesion of the TCCG: its sensitivity in the literature is well recognised, varying from 89% to 95% depending on the series (37).

However, the specificity of this test in detecting lesions of the TCCG is debated.

3. Myocardial scintigraphy data :

Myocardial scintigraphy is highly effective in detecting lesions of the TCCG. Its sensitivity is high, ranging from 60 to 92% depending on the author (38).

The specific abnormality of a lesion of the TCCG during myocardial scintigraphy is localised hypo-fixation at the level of the septum, the anterior wall and the lateral wall.

However, in all the series in the literature, there are a few cases of normal myocardial scintigraphy (39).

Chikamori (38) in a series of 466 patients with CGRT stenosis, proposed four scintigraphic anomalies as highly suggestive of a CGRT lesion:

- Fixation anomalies
- Slow, diffuse washing of thalium
- Presence of ischaemia
- Diffuse perfusion disorders

4. Echocardiographic data :

Visualisation of the left LADC by two-dimensional echocardiography has been studied by many authors.

It is possible to identify a stenosis of the TCCG using TTE without coronary angiography, but this examination has many limitations in the positive diagnosis of stenoses of the TCCG.

The sensitivity of this test is far from satisfactory (60%) (40).

As a result, this examination is of no practical value in the search for lesions of the TCCG.

Some authors have studied the velocity of diastolic flow by pulsed Doppler at the level of the TCCG in short axis paraspinal section as markers of significant stenosis of the TCCG (40) (32) . An acceleration in diastolic flow velocity above 112 m/s is an indication of significant stenosis of the CSGC.

Visualisation of stenoses of the TCCG is easier with TEE than with TTE (41). Colour Doppler flow analysis can be used to assess the severity of lesions of the LCCT on TEE.

The sensitivity of TEE in detecting tight lesions of the TCCG is 91% with a specificity of 100%, the positive predictive value is 100% and the negative predictive value is 98% when the TCCG is properly visualised. However, its value in the study of lesions of the TCCG is debated by several authors who report less concordant results between TEE and coronary angiography in cases of poorly assessed eccentric stenosis, in the presence of calcifications and because of the difficulty of distinguishing between stenosis and sinuosity. (42).

5. Coronary CT data :

The multi-slice scanner (MSS) is an interesting, safe and promising non-invasive coronary imaging technique. The current generation of 64-slice scanners uses a high resolution of 0.4 mm with thin sections of 0.6 mm and a temporal resolution of 165 ms, and the simultaneous acquisition of 64 parallel sections, enabling visualisation of the entire coronary tree in less than 10 seconds. (43) (44).

In the literature, coroscans are of excellent value in the diagnosis of significant lesions of the small arteries, with 86 to 94% sensitivity and 93 to 97% specificity (45).

However, the 64-slice scanner comes up against a number of problems when assessing stenoses in the TCCG.

Kuettner and Juwana (46) pointed out in their studies that BMS detects lesions but underestimates them. This underestimation is mainly due to calcifications.

Calcifications are the main cause of error in reading and interpreting the data provided by the SMB.

6. Coronary angiography data :

Coronary angiography remains the gold standard for the diagnosis of stenosis of the TCCG (47).

This examination enables an anatomical description of the lesion to be made, its location to be determined, its extent to be determined, and the extent of any associated coronary lesions to be assessed.

These parameters are important in the therapeutic decision, making it possible, in association with the other clinical and ultrasound data, to direct the therapeutic indications towards an interventional or surgical alternative.

Given the seriousness of the complications that can arise during coronography or in the hours that follow, certain precautions must be taken:

- Use non-invasive tests to look for evidence of a lesion of the TCCG.

- Perform an initial non-selective injection in the coronary sinus to detect predominantly ostial involvement of the TCCG.

- Avoid "jumping" the probe in the TCCG and advance the probe carefully and slowly through the TCCG.

- Strictly check the pressure at the end of the probe and the electrical aspect before and after each injection.

- Ensure safe reflux into the sinus of Valsalva.

- Shorten the procedure to obtain as much information as possible with the least possible injections and the lowest possible volume of contrast medium.

- The injection of the contrast product must be gentle and must avoid injections with strong pressure.

6. 1. Location of stenosis :

The study of the GCCT can be difficult for lesions that are ostial, proximal, distal and extending to the anterior interventricular-circumflex bifurcation.

All the authors have noted the vast majority of distal location. Indeed, Seung (31) reported a distal location in 51% of cases, while Cheng (23) reported a distal location in 61.1% of cases.

The ostial location of a significant CGRT lesion appears to be rarer and more frequent in women (48) (16).

Some studies have concluded that the prevalence of ostial and intermediate lesions of the TCCG varies from 19% to 51%. (49) (50) (31) (51).

Angiographic exploration of the literature has shown that the distal site of the TCCG lesion is the most frequent location, with a rate of distal TCCG lesions that varies from 51% in the MAIN COMPARE study (31) study to 72% in the Boudriot (22).

Table II shows the location of stenosis of the TCCG according to the different studies.

Table II: Locations of stenosis of the TCCG.

	Ostial /proximal	Median	distal
Boudriot (22)	20 %	6 %	74 %
Lee (29)	38,9%		61 %

6. 2. Degree of stenosis :

The severity of CGRT stenosis varies according to coronary angiography series (47).

Stenoses are usually classified into 3 stages according to their severity:

Stage I: 50% to 69

Stage II: 70% to 89

Stage III: > 90

Most authors agree that stage I predominates, with percentages of the order of 51% to 80%, and that stage III does not exceed 30% of all narrowings of the TCCG (52) (53).

Table III gives an idea of the percentages of each group in two different studies:

Table III: Distribution of patients according to the degree of stenosis of the TCCG .

	Rollé (54)	Carrié (55)
Stage I	42 %	60 %
Stage II	37 %	30 %
Stage III	21 %	10 %

6. 3. Associated lesions :

Damage to the TCCG is most often associated with damage to other coronary arteries. It seems to indicate diffuse and severe atherosclerotic disease. These are frequently tri-truncular lesions (11) (16).

Analysis of the coronary status of patients from different series revealed that involvement of the TCCG was associated with other coronary lesions in all cases, with a clear predominance of tri-truncular status (31) (56).

In the SYNTAX study (56), a fairly high proportion of isolated stenosis of the TCCG and mono-truncular involvement were noted.

Table IV summarises the coronary status in certain series.

Table IV: Coronary lesions associated with stenosis of the TCCG .

	Lee et al (29)	Boudriot (22)	Cheng (23)	SYNTAX study (56)
Isolated TCCG	17%	28%	15%	13 %
Monotruncular disease	22,6%	32%	16%	15 %
Bi-truncular disease	31%	27%	22%	26 %
Tri-truncular involvement	29, %	13%	47%	46 %

6. 4. Isolated ostial stenosis of the TCCG :

Isolated ostial stenosis of the TCCG is a special entity, characterised by its rarity and the particular profile of patients with this type of stenosis.

Arima (59) showed that isolated ostial damage to the TCCG occurs mainly in pre-menopausal women who have a low incidence of coronary risk factors. The author explains that this type of TCCG lesion is not due solely to atheromatous disease but also to other factors such as vasospasm and aortic inflammatory disease.

From a technical point of view, the angiographic diagnosis of this type of lesion is sometimes difficult to establish. The operator may selectively intubate the TCCG without paying attention to the ostium, thus obtaining a normal coronary network. For this reason, non-selective injections are recommended in order to visualise the ostial TCCG.

6.5 Chronic occlusion of the TCCG :

Chronic occlusion of the TCCG is a rare entity. Its incidence varies between 0.02% and 0.7 (60).

The progressive development of lesions on the TCCG probably helps to explain the development of a good collaterality ensuring survival and the preservation of good left ventricular function. (61).

Thus, three conditions are essential for survival and the preservation of good left ventricular function in patients with chronic occlusion of the TCCG: dominance of the right network, the presence of well-developed collaterality, and the absence of lesions in the right coronary network. (62).

7. Data from the IVUS (intravascular ultrasound study) :

The use of IVUS to assess lesions of the TCCG has become an important diagnostic element.

It enables a highly detailed, high-resolution cross-sectional study of the coronary arteries to be carried out in vivo. It also makes it possible to study the architecture of the coronary arterial wall, the composition of the atherosclerotic plaque, and the changes in the arterial wall secondary to the progression of atherosclerotic disease. (63).

Several studies have investigated the threshold at which a lesion of the TCCG is considered to be tight. Gil (64) showed that the most reliable parameter is the minimum luminal diameter. If the minimum luminal diameter is ≤ 2 mm, the probability of a significant lesion of the TCCG is high.

8. FFR (fractional flow reserve) data :

This is an invasive examination that studies coronary perfusion in a functional way. The value of FFR calculated from the measurement of pressures in the coronary arteries has been shown to be a sensitive and specific index for determining whether a coronary lesion is significant in functional terms and whether it is responsible for myocardial ischaemia (65).

The presence of lesions in the TCCG can have major therapeutic implications: the degree of stenosis in the TCCG has a direct influence on the indications for treatment, whether medical, surgical or interventional.

In practice, however, there are patients with angiographically moderate stenoses of the TCCG in whom the therapeutic decision is often difficult. In fact, these patients may have significant lesions in terms of function and are therefore exposed to a significant risk of morbidity and mortality.

On the other hand, when aorto-coronary bypass surgery is indicated and carried out in the event of overestimation of these lesions in the TCCG, this leads to inappropriate use of arterial or venous grafts and premature occlusion of the native vessels.

Bech (65) in a study including 57 patients with intermediate lesions of the TCCG, showed that 56% of patients with a stenosis angiographically estimated at 40 to 60% actually had a lesion judged to be tight by FFR (FFR < 0.75). In this study, these patients (FFR < 0.75) underwent coronary artery bypass grafting, while the other patients (FFR $\geq$ 0.75) received medical treatment. The results after 3 years of follow-up showed excellent survival for both groups, although the angiographic diameters of the TCCG were comparable.

V- Therapeutic management :

The treatment of stenosis of the TCCG is based on 3 components: a medical component, a surgical component and an interventional component.

Medical treatment is essential and should be started as soon as possible after patients are admitted to hospital. However, treatment alone is insufficient.

For a long time, surgery was considered to be the fundamental treatment for CGRT stenosis. The development of surgical techniques and means of myocardial protection has greatly improved surgical results and short-, medium- and long-term prognosis.

Interventional treatment has now become an important therapeutic component, especially following the development of active stents and the associated revolution in pharmacological treatment.

The treatment of chronic occlusion of the TCCG is essentially surgical. Coronary artery bypass grafting has the best results in terms of morbidity and mortality compared with medical treatment (66).

1. *Medical treatment :*

Medical treatment plays an important role in the management of CGRT stenosis. This treatment is always combined with surgical or interventional treatment.

Medical treatment alone is associated with greater morbidity and mortality than surgical or interventional treatment.

Indeed, several early clinical trials have demonstrated a survival benefit of coronary artery bypass grafting compared with medical treatment alone (67) (19).

For example, in the CASS study, survival at 3 years for the surgical group was 91% compared with 69% for the medical group; at 4 years these figures had risen to 88% and 63% respectively. (19).

At present, medical treatment alone is indicated for :

- Inoperable patients, due to the presence of diffuse and distal coronary lesions with a poor downstream bed and/or very severe impairment of LVEF, or inoperable due to associated extra-cardiac conditions with a poor prognosis.

- Patients who are operable but have refused surgery.

2. Surgical revascularisation :

Surgical revascularisation of CGRT stenosis has been shown to be effective in improving survival rates and quality of life for patients undergoing surgery.

1. 1. Operating time (68) :

In the majority of cases, patients with CGRT stenosis are operated on rapidly, except in cases of extreme emergency.

Several authors have studied the evolution of these patients in the days leading up to the operation in order to determine the factors with a poor prognosis and to identify the indications for urgent surgery.

Maziak et al (69) concluded that surgery should be performed within the first 10 days of catheterisation in patients with severe symptoms or recent myocardial infarction.

Da Rocha (70) showed that patients presenting with a tight stenosis of the TCCG whose reason for discovery was acute coronary syndrome have a risk of cardiovascular events five times greater than other clinical presentations, even after the patient has stabilised clinically. This author indicated that patients admitted for acute coronary syndrome in connection with a tight stenosis of the TCCG should be given special attention and should be operated on as soon as possible.

Preoperative haemodynamic instability in the Murzi study (71) is a poor prognostic factor.

1. 2. Approach :

The classic approach currently used by most surgeons is the median sternotomy. This allows rapid and easy installation of the bypass graft, good visualisation of the coronary arteries and easy dislocation of the heart to allow coronary anastomoses to be made correctly (Figure 1).

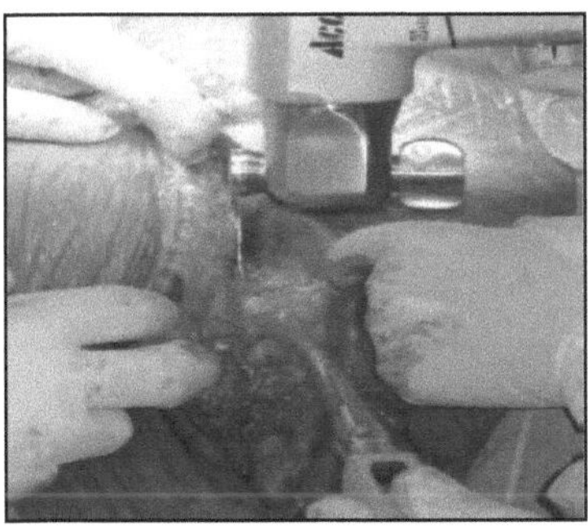

Figure 1: Vertical median sternotomy .

In many specialities, surgery has gradually evolved towards less invasive techniques in order to limit parietal trauma. The decisive step was undoubtedly the use of video-assisted techniques for totally endoscopic surgery, which has become the reference technique in certain specialities. In coronary artery bypass surgery, because of the impossibility of performing microsurgical sutures using two-dimensional endoscopic vision, the concept of minimally invasive surgery initially sought to do away with the need for extracorporeal circulation (ECG) with the development of off-pump coronary artery bypass techniques (OPCAB) performed in most cases by median sternotomy.

Subsequently, the use of video-assisted surgery has made it possible to develop limited thoracic approaches combining video-assisted harvesting of the left internal mammary pedicle and direct-view coronary anastomosis by left mini-thoracotomy: either with a beating heart using the MIDCAB (mini invasive direct coronary artery bypass) technique, or with a stopped heart under femoral bypass using the port-access technique (Figure 2).

The approach was a left anterior mini-thoracotomy in the 5ème intercostal space.

These techniques have their own limitations: the MIDCAB technique can only be used to perform a single breast implant on the IVA; coronary multi-bridges are theoretically accessible to the port-access technique, but in reality they are difficult to perform, particularly when two breast pedicles are used.

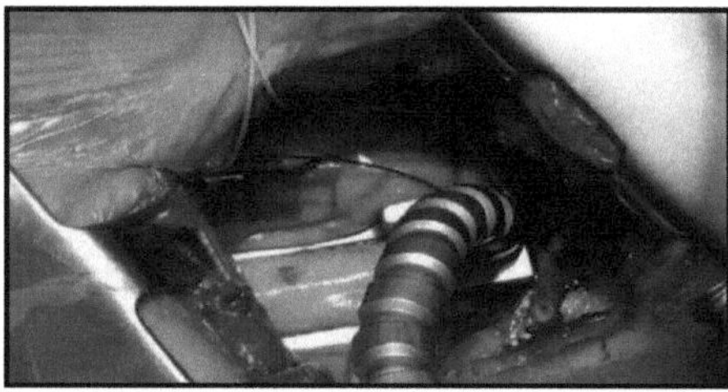

Figure 2: Intraoperative image of a coronary bypass using the MIDCAB technique.

The advantage of the robotic remote manipulator is that it enables the surgeon's vision and both hands to be transferred virtually and with the chest closed, right in contact with the tissues. The contribution of the robotic technique in coronary surgery is therefore an important step forward, since it allows coronary anastomoses to be performed completely endoscopically, thanks to three-dimensional vision and instruments adapted to microsurgery (72). The robotic remote manipulator must be considered above all as a tool whose use is subject to a minimum of prerequisites, such as experience in video surgery and coronary surgery without extracorporeal circulation.

Thanks to the robotic remote manipulator, the various stages of coronary surgery can be carried out completely endoscopically: removal of the mammary pedicles, pericardotomy, control of the coronaries, and anastomoses (73).

Its use allows video-assisted breast harvesting to be optimised without question, and it is essential for harvesting both breast pedicles through the same hemi-thorax.

Coronary bypass surgery can therefore be carried out either with the heart beating without bypass grafting, with the heart beating under bypass grafting, or with the heart stopped under bypass grafting.

1. 3. Coronary artery bypass graft :

Aorto-coronary bypass surgery is the standard treatment for myocardial revascularisation. The principle is based on creating a bridge between the aorta and the coronary artery downstream of the stenosis.

A mammary artery is almost always used. In multiple bypasses, the choice of other grafts is vast, ranging from the long saphenous vein to the radial artery and the gastroepiploic artery.

The frequency of coronary lesions associated with stenosis of the TCCG implies a high number of bypasses per patient, on average between 2.6 and 3.1 bypasses per patient (54). In Holm's study of 330 patients (9), 1001 bypasses were placed, corresponding to an average of 3 bypasses per patient. Left mammary bypass was performed in 258 patients (78%), arterial bypass in only 5. In only one case was the gastroepiploic artery used. The remainder were venous bypasses.

Several teams are currently performing an all-arterial bypass using either the two internal mammary arteries, a sequential arterial bypass, or both procedures at the same time. Venous grafts are increasingly being abandoned because of the rapid degeneration of these bridges.

*** 1. 4. Endarterectomy with TCCG widening plasty :*

This is an old surgical technique dating back to 1965 when Effler and Sabiston (74) (75) performed a surgical reconstruction of the ostium of the TCCG.

The principle is to remove the atheromatous plaque with the endartery and enlarge the ostium with a patch. This procedure should be carried out if there is good left ventricular function and no calcifications, and requires a correct approach to the trunk by moving the trunk away from the pulmonary artery.

This technique restores physiological anterograde flow in the coronary arteries, which is theoretically better than retrograde perfusion by conventional bypass surgery. The internal mammary artery and saphenous vein capital are preserved by this technique, and percutaneous trans-luminal coronary angioplasty of distal coronary lesions is always possible (76).

The first enlargement patches were venous or pericardial and gave good results despite the high risk of restenosis, due to the properties of the venous patch, which degenerated rapidly, or that of the pericardium, which could calcify.

Martinovic (77), in a series of 37 patients, showed that surgical reconstruction of the TCCG with an autologous patch is an effective and safe technique for treating ostial and proximal stenosis of the TCCG. In this series, there was no mortality and no major complications. During the follow-up period (3 years on average), only one patient presented with a coronary syndrome, for which coronary angiography showed significant distal stenosis of the TCCG at the level of the terminal part of the enlargement patch. This author proposed only isolated, ostial and proximal stenosis of the TCCG in the absence of severe calcifications as indications for surgical reconstruction of the TCCG.

Maureira (78), in a larger study including 97 patients who had undergone TCCG plasty, reported an overall mortality of 95% at 5 years and 80% at 10 years.

In 2015, a study published by BERNAL et al (79) concluded that coronary artery endarterectomy in patients with a high or intermediate EuroSCORE reduces morbidity and mortality, which leads us to think about it in high-risk patients.

Another recent study published in 2016 found that this revascularisation technique is not associated with a higher rate of post-operative mortality and morbidity than bypass revascularisation (80).

1. 5. Beating heart bypass :

Coronary bypass surgery under CEC allows surgeons to better expose the heart and perform very complicated technical procedures. However, the use of CEC is associated with certain complications such as myocardial ischaemia, stroke, post-operative neuro-cognitive disorders, renal failure, transfusions and supra-ventricular rhythm disorders.

In order to prevent these complications, surgeons have returned to beating heart surgery, particularly following the current improvements in surgical techniques, anaesthetic procedures and post-operative resuscitation.

Revascularisation surgery without CEC, in cases of stenosis of the TCCG, is a safe alternative to surgery under CEC (81) (82).

Robert (81) compared 420 patients who underwent beating heart surgery with 234 patients who underwent bypass surgery. He found that the time to overall ischaemia was shorter, the incidence of blood transfusion and renal failure, and the use of intra-aortic counterpulsation postoperatively were lower in the case of beating heart surgery. In addition, operative mortality was significantly lower in the beating heart group (1.9%), compared with 6.4% in the bypass group.

This beating heart surgery has significantly reduced the frequency of rhythm disorders, renal complications, transfusions and neurological complications (83) (5).

These advantages have made this technique widely used throughout the world. In fact, beating heart CABG is performed in 20% of cases in the USA, 15% in Canada and up to 85% of cases in Chinese centres (84).

However, the beating heart surgical treatment of tight lesions of the TCCG was at one time considered to be a relative contraindication, in relation to the haemodynamic disturbances that occur when the heart is dislocated during this surgical procedure.

Nowadays, haemodynamic disturbances have been improved by technological advances and better anaesthetic techniques and procedures, making this method of revascularisation safer.

Several authors (85) (81) have shown that beating heart TCCG surgery is a safe method, effective in terms of early and late mortality, and in terms of cardiovascular events. This technique has also given satisfactory results for patients with left ventricular dysfunction (86).

In a comparative study between beating heart surgery and angioplasty of the TCCG using active stents, the difference in operative mortality and neurological complications was not significant. But the difference in hospital MACE between the two groups was significant (0.94% in the angioplasty group versus 5.78% in the bypass group, with p < 0.05). However, the difference in MACE after 12 months' follow-up was not significant (3.77% in the angioplasty group versus 3.31% in the beating heart surgery group and p > 0.05) (87). This technique therefore requires more randomised studies in order to assess its benefit in the postoperative period, and to refine the indications for this procedure in cases of isolated involvement of the TCCG, and associated mono- or multi-truncular involvement.

However, conversion from beating heart surgery to bypass surgery is always possible. In a multivariate analysis, pulmonary hypertension and mitral regurgitation were predictive of conversion (88). In-hospital mortality was 3.2% for patients who underwent beating heart surgery and 9% for patients who underwent conventional surgery. This study (89) concluded that beating heart surgery has better results for high-risk patients, i.e. patients with severe CKGR stenosis, acute coronary syndrome with persistent resting chest pain, unstable angina, ventricular arrhythmia or impaired LVEF.

Another treatment option for coronary artery disease patients with CGRT stenosis and a high surgical risk is integrated coronary revascularisation, or hybrid revascularisation according to some authors.

This method of revascularisation combines the breast bypass technique with angioplasty. In this procedure, the surgeon performs a minimally invasive direct breast bypass via a left thoracotomy without extracorporeal circulation. Then, within a week, the angio-plastician performs an angioplasty of the distal branches of the circumflex artery and/or the right coronary artery (90) (91).

This type of revascularisation does not improve the rate of early survival, but it does reduce the length of hospital stay in intensive care units, the duration of mechanical ventilation, the need for blood transfusions, and reduces hospital costs (92).

This method could therefore be highly effective in the hands of angio-plasticians in high-volume centres (more than 600 angioplasties per year) and surgeons experienced in breast bypass surgery without extra-corporeal circulation.

However, most of the series published in the literature reported on small groups of patients treated with a maximum follow-up of 1 year.

1. 6. Combined CABG and aortic valve replacement surgery :

The incidence of coronary artery disease is excessively high in patients with aortic stenosis. This frequency varies from region to region, but above all with age: around 40% before the age of 60, and up to 60% after the age of 80 (93) (94).

Operative mortality is doubled in the case of coronary revascularisation associated with valve replacement (95) (96) (97) (98).

1. 7. Coronary surgery and carotid thromboendarterectomy :

Evagelopoulos et al (65) have shown that in the case of association of significant stenosis of the TCCG with lesions of the internal carotid artery, combined surgery of carotid endarterectomy and myocardial revascularisation is justified, and that the risk of MI and stroke is no greater than in the case of isolated surgery of each lesion.

Beating heart coronary surgery reduces the risk of neurological complications in patients with significant carotid stenosis and a history of stroke.

However, large-scale studies are needed to confirm these results (99).

VI- Results of surgery :

Several studies have analysed mortality, complications and major events in the short, medium and long term, depending on the surgical technique and patient profile.

1. Operative mortality :

In-hospital and out-of-hospital operative mortality were analysed at the same time, as only one patient died during the out-of-hospital phase in our series.

Since the early days of coronary revascularisation surgery, stenosis of the TCCG has been recognised as a peri-operative risk factor in its own right (19).

Over the last few decades, the risk inherent in this particular pathology has diminished but has not disappeared (100) (101).

This improvement in results is secondary to the development of microsurgical techniques, myocardial protection, anaesthesia and, above all, the use of arterial grafts.

In 1997, the registry of the Society of Thoracic Surgery reported an operative risk of 4% in patients with stenosis of the TCCG, i.e. a risk 1.5 times higher than for all coronary surgeries (4 versus 2.5%). (102).

Recent series have found an intra-hospital mortality rate of 2.8% and a 30-day mortality rate of between 3 and 4.2%, similar to that for coronary surgery in general (71) (103).

The mortality rate increases with the number of coronary trunks affected. In the SYNTAX study, the mortality rates at 1, 2, 3 and 5 years for severe multitruncular disease were 3.5%, 4.9%, 6.7% and 11.4% **respectively** (57) (58).

2. Different predictive scores for operative mortality :

The early post-operative period is classically recognised as being the most critical, and attempts are therefore being made to determine the prognostic factors predictive of early mortality.

Several scores are currently used to estimate operative mortality in cardiac surgery.

The aim of risk scores in cardiac surgery is to estimate operative mortality (at 30 days) after cardiac surgery, depending on the patient's characteristics and the type of surgery. They therefore play an important role in estimating the risk/benefit ratio of operations and in patient information. The scores discriminate fairly well between low-risk and high-risk patients. However, they lack precision when it comes to estimating mortality figures, and the EuroSCORE in particular tends to overestimate operative mortality, the higher the risk.

Risk scores therefore have the advantage of reducing the subjectivity of operative risk assessment, but they must be interpreted with caution and cannot replace clinical judgement.

Certain factors (PURSUIT risk score) have also been identified by certain studies as being predictive of an increase in perioperative mortality (104).

EuroSCORE was developed by the European Association of Cardio-Thoracic Surgery. It is a single score for all types of cardiac surgery.

It is widely used, not least because it is so easy to use. The additive version can be calculated at the patient's bedside by simple addition. The logistic version enables the probability of perioperative death to be estimated directly, but requires a calculator. EuroSCORE II is currently used. Various parameters are being studied.

The STS score is derived from the Society of Thoracic Surgeons database. It includes a larger number of variables than the EuroSCORE, and therefore takes longer to calculate. It has the advantage of including specific models for the different types of cardiac surgery (valvular or coronary or other) and estimates not only operative mortality but also morbidity.

In addition to the SYNTAX anatomical score and the SYNTAX clinical score, Farooq et al (92) have developed the SYNTAX score II, which contains 8 parameters and predicts 4-year mortality in patients with complex coronary lesions.

3. Clinical factors :

Diabetes is a factor that worsens the prognosis of post-operative patients through mediastinal and pulmonary infections, as well as the metabolic disorders it causes.

The percentage of diabetics was 14.4% in the series by Lu et al (103)and 19% in the study by Murzi (71).

Several studies, such as those by Murzi (71) and Ellis (105), have identified diabetes as being responsible for excess mortality. A recent study by YU et al (17) found that diabetes did not influence mortality or the occurrence of postoperative MI or stroke. In the BARI and FREEDOM study (106) (107)diabetic and multitruncular patients who underwent coronary artery bypass grafting (CABG) had greater survival than patients who underwent TKA.

Age increases the risk of surgery. In the CASS study (19), the operative mortality rate increased proportionally with age, rising from 2% in patients under 50 to 7% after 50 (p=0.002). Age has also been identified as a predictive factor in studies by Lu (103), Murzi (71), Ellis (105) and YU (68).

Joseph (108) in a study including 3083 patients with stenosis of the TCCG, showed that advanced age is an important factor in early mortality (p < 0.0001) (108). However, Rollé (54) reported only 3% death in 50 patients with CGRT stenosis aged over 70 years.

Female gender is a risk factor for surgery (102). In the CASS (19)study, operative mortality was estimated at 8% in women versus 4% in men (p=0.02). This excess mortality rate in women has been noted in other studies: Gomberg (109)in a retrospective post-operative study of 176 patients operated on for common trunk stenosis, found the same findings, noting a mortality rate of 6.6% in men and 17.5% in women (p<0.05). It has also been reported that the overall increase in the percentage of women recognised as having unfavourable anatomical conditions with a smaller coronary diameter than men is more significant in the age groups over 60 and 70 years (110).

Several studies have attempted to assess the impact of clinical presentation on mortality and the occurrence of MACE.

The risk increases with the clinical severity of functional impairment. In Chaitman's study (111)patients suffering from acute coronary syndrome had a higher operative mortality rate (6%) than patients with stable angina (3%).

Da Rocha (70) showed that patients presenting with a tight stenosis of the TCCG whose reason for discovery was an acute coronary syndrome have a risk of cardiovascular events 5 times greater than other clinical presentations, even after the patient's clinical stabilisation.

Fuikui et al (88) in a study of 459 patients, 191 of whom had an acute coronary syndrome as their clinical presentation, demonstrated that this clinical presentation had no impact either in the short or long term on mortality or on the occurrence of MACE. (15).

Patients hospitalised for myocardial infarction are at greater risk of peri- and post-operative mortality than other patients (54).

Left ventricular dysfunction is one of the complications of coronary artery disease, and is a risk factor in patients with ischaemic heart disease proposed for coronary artery bypass surgery. Despite advances in new therapeutic classes, interventional cardiology and surgical techniques, in-hospital mortality in patients with impaired left ventricular function remains high compared with patients with preserved LV function (112).

Heart failure associated with a profound deterioration in ventricular ejection fraction is a highly predictive factor of peri-operative mortality (8% mortality versus 4% in the absence of heart failure according to the CASS study). (19).

- Association with peripheral vascular disease :

In the literature, the association with atherosclerotic disease of the peripheral arteries has been described, and has been judged to be a factor that increases the mortality rate by 25% compared with patients with associated coronary disease (31).

- Chronic renal failure :

Renal failure has been identified as a prognostic factor for in-hospital mortality in several studies, such as the Ellis study (105).

In a recent study published by Pan et al in 2016 (113)patients with CKGR stenosis who have normal renal function or a clearance greater than 45 ml/min, TCA is a good alternative to surgery. However, for patients with severe renal function (cl <45 ml / min $\times$ 1.73 m^2), patients have a high risk of myocardial infarction after the procedure.

In a multivariate analysis, pre-operative chronic renal failure was strongly correlated with in-hospital mortality (p = 0.006).

- Acute postoperative renal failure :

In a multi-centre study of 2222 patients, the aim of which was to assess renal dysfunction after coronary artery bypass grafting under CEC, renal dysfunction was defined as a creatinine level greater than or equal to 20 mg/l, or an increase of 7 mg/l or more compared with the pre-operative level. (114). Renal dysfunction occurred in 7.7% of patients, and 1.4% required haemodialysis sessions. In-hospital mortality was 19% in the group that did not use haemodialysis pre-operatively, and 63% in the group that did, compared with a mortality rate of 0.9% in patients who were free of renal dysfunction.

4. *Coronary factors :*

The CASS study (19) study demonstrated the influence of the severity of the MCCT lesion: 50-74% MCCT involvement had no effect on mortality (2.1% versus 2.3%). When trunk involvement is < 75%, dominance does not influence prognosis. However, if the involvement is severe >90%, mortality increases from 5.7% for right dominance to 25% for left dominance.

Involvement of the right coronary artery, especially when it is dominant, is also a key prognostic factor, and many authors agree that the time and type of surgery should be determined by the degree of compensation of the right coronary artery. (115) (116). Isolated ostial location is not correlated with an increase in operative morbidity and mortality (16).

JONSSON (92), compared early and late mortality after coronary trunk surgery in patients who did not have a stenosis of the TCCG, in patients who had an intermediate stenosis of less than 75%, in patients who had a severe stenosis of more than 75%, and in patients who had an occlusion of the TCCG.

These patients were followed for 10 years. Early mortality was 1.9% and 2.3% respectively in the absence or presence of intermediate stenosis, compared with 6.3% if the stenosis was severe. Survival at 10 years was 76% in the absence of stenosis of the TCCG, 74% in the presence of intermediate stenosis and 64% in the presence of severe stenosis. (13).

In the SYNTAX (117)study, the incidence of death and myocardial infarction was 2.1% in the case of isolated involvement of the left coronary trunk, 7.4 to 7.7% in the case of involvement of the GTCT with 1 vessel and involvement of the GTCT with 2 vessels, and increased significantly to 14.5% in the case of involvement of the GTCT with 3 vessels.

5. Surgical factors :

- **Operative delay:** Because of the risk of complications, it is advisable to operate on patients with CGRT stenosis relatively soon after coronary angiography. Ideally, the operation should be performed during the same hospital stay.

The circumstances of the operation also have a definite prognostic value. Emergency surgery performed in poor conditions of haemodynamic instability and acute necrosis is associated with a high mortality rate (up to 40%). In fact, for practical reasons, these patients should be scheduled on a semi-emergency basis, with the time taken adapted to each individual case.

Holm (9) found a high mortality rate in emergency surgery performed in poor conditions of cardiovascular instability and myocardial ischaemia, since 79% of patients who died were in the emergency surgery group. This author recommended stabilisation of myocardial ischaemia and haemodynamic status prior to surgery.

It is therefore advisable, except in cases of extreme urgency, to wait a reasonable amount of time before handing the patient over to the surgeons in the best possible conditions.

Maziak et al (69) recommended meticulous selection of patients with CKGR stenosis, and advised urgent surgery (less than 10 days) in subjects with severe symptoms. acute coronary syndrome or pre-operative MI, or rest dyspnoea.

However, for a stenosis exceeding 75% of the TCCG, the operative delay can be extended to 3 weeks in clinically stabilised subjects.

Similarly, Rexius H (118) found that emergency procedures had a significantly higher mortality than elective procedures and that triage based primarily on clinical symptomatology, and secondarily on the degree of stenosis, must be well established.

- **Intra-operative myocardial protection:** The quality of myocardial protection determines the post-operative prognosis. The cardioplegia solution must stop the heart, protect it and provide it with the elements it needs to survive until it resumes its activity. It must preserve its ATP reserves and intracellular enzymes, minimise anaerobic metabolism, and prevent the formation of free radicals and calcium overload during reperfusion.

Deviri et al (119) prefer warm blood cardioplegia for better myocardial protection in patients with CGRT stenosis.

Retrograde cardioplegia via the coronary sinus has the advantage of reaching distal territories in the case of proximal tight stenoses with little collateralisation, and of avoiding aortic leakage, but it does not protect the right ventricle, whose drainage is via the veins of Thebesius and not via the coronary sinus. The cannula is inserted by puncturing the right atrium; it has a semi-occlusive cuff. Perfusion pressure must remain between 30 and 40 mm Hg, and is measured by a separate pressure transducer. The flow rate is 100-200 ml/min.

- **Duration of aortic clamping and extra-corporeal circulation:** The duration of aortic clamping and extra-corporeal circulation are very important factors in operative and post-operative mortality. In fact, the longer these durations are, the greater the mortality. (102).

Chaitman (111) reported in his series of 1172 patients undergoing surgery that the duration of extracorporeal circulation was longer in non-survivors (156 ± 62 versus 118 ± 45 minutes; $p < 0.0001$). More recently,

Rollé (120) showed that mortality in the early post-operative period was statistically correlated with a duration of extra-corporeal circulation greater than 140 minutes and an aortic clamping time greater than 100 minutes.

Table V summarises the duration of bypass surgery and aortic clamping in a number of series in the literature.

Table V: Summary table of the duration of CEC and aortic clamping in certain series.

series	Year	Duration of CEC (min)	Duration of aortic clamping (min)
Sheri Murtaza M (121)	2009	111,53	64,07
Chaitman (111)	1983	137+/-53	-
Deviri (119)	1993	141 ± 39.55	73.03 ± 17.96

- Complete or incomplete myocardial revascularisation and the number of aorto-coronary bypasses: Incomplete revascularisation is an important prognostic factor, as it exposes the patient to early post-operative infarction and impairment of ejection fraction.

Nataf (122) showed that incomplete revascularisation is an independent factor in peri-operative mortality (p < 0.005). In a study including 3803 patients who had undergone CABG for tight stenosis of the TCCG, incomplete revascularisation was a factor in post-operative morbidity and a factor in subsequent re intervention (108).

Rollé (54) also emphasised the detrimental effect of incomplete revascularisation. However, some authors believe that the degree of revascularisation may be more important in terms of long-term survival and functional results than in the immediate term.

The type and number of grafts used can also have an impact on post-operative results. In fact, the use of 2 breast grafts is associated with a lower risk than the use of a saphenous graft, occlusion of which is more frequent postoperatively than arterial grafts (p = 0.008). (122).

Joseph (108) showed that the use of the internal mammary artery as a graft on the IVA or the diagonal or both at the same time significantly improved survival (p=0.003). The number of bridges is also a prognostic factor since it is generally dependent on complete revascularisation, with 10% of deaths observed when the number of bridges is < 2 versus 4% if the number of bridges is ≥ 2.

- **Length of mechanical ventilation and length of stay in intensive care:** Lu et al (103) demonstrated that the duration of mechanical ventilation exceeding 48 hours and a stay in an intensive care unit were not predictive factors of mortality. However, a total length of stay exceeding 14 days was significantly predictive of mortality, hence the advantage of beating heart surgery.

6. *Post-operative morbidity :*

In series published in the literature, postoperative MI is slightly more frequent than during coronary surgery in general. While the rate of such a complication is 2 to 10% in coronary surgery (123)it appears to be twice as high for common trunk stenosis surgery. The factors determining the occurrence of post-operative ischaemic complications in patients with acute occlusion of the TCCG are haemodynamic status, the presence or absence of collateral circulation, the success of coronary reperfusion and the presence of a dominant right coronary network (124).

In the SYNTAX study, the rate of stroke after CABG for TCCG stenosis was 4.3% in patients who underwent surgery, compared with 1.5% in patients who underwent percutaneous angioplasty (p = 0.03). (125).

7. Late results :

Surgical treatment of CGRT stenosis by aorto-coronary bypass has also transformed the vital and functional prognosis of patients in the medium and long term.

The CASS study (19) studied the follow-up of patients over a period of 15, 11 and 10 years respectively, showing a clear increase in survival compared with medical treatment, with a 15-year survival rate of 37%. The greater the degree of stenosis in the trunk, the greater the benefit.

Joseph (108) reported a 10-year survival of 64% and a 20-year survival of 28%. This author reported several factors predictive of medium- and long-term mortality: left ventricular dysfunction, diabetes, hypertension, peripheral arterial disease, smoking, use of venous grafts and pre-operative atrial fibrillation.

Cardiovascular causes of late death include heart failure, sudden death, MI, and rhythm or conduction disorders. (126). This secondary mortality is much lower than the spontaneous mortality of this type of patient, since it is accepted that almost half of non-operated patients die within 3 years of coronary angiography. Surgery therefore unquestionably increases the life expectancy of these patients.

Table VI shows the operative and long-term mortality of coronary artery bypass grafting:

Table VI: Coronary artery bypass grafting for CAGT stenosis: in-hospital and out-of-hospital mortality .

Author	Year of study	Year of surgery	Number of patients	Mortality	
				Hospital %	Outpatient %
Jonsson (77)	2006	1970-99	1888	2,7	-
Lu (103)	2005	1997-2003	1197	2,8	10
Keogh and kinsman (78)	2003	2003	5003	3	-
Dewey (122)	2006	1998-99	728	-	4,2
Yeatman (79)	2006	1996-2000	387	2,4	-
Joseph (108)	2006	1971-98	3803	-	7,8

The improved survival of patients who have undergone surgery is accompanied by improved function, since 70-90% of survivors are asymptomatic after a follow-up of up to 5 years (55).

Carrie et al (55) recorded the functional status at 18 months of 134 patients with a significant lesion of the TCCG, and found a clear functional improvement in the surgically revascularised group.

VII- Surgery versus angioplasty in the management of unprotected TCCG lesions:

Stenosis of the unprotected TCCG, the most severe of coronary lesions because of the large myocardial territory affected by ischaemia, has benefited since 1995 from an alternative to coronary surgery with the introduction of stenting of the common trunk in carefully selected cases.

In the presence of involvement of the TCCG, coronary revascularisation by bypass surgery was the rule for several years, based in part on the CASS (19). It was suggested that certain pathophysiological characteristics militated against the success of angioplasty, namely the high risk of re-stenosis in the presence of a bifurcation lesion and the fact that the majority of patients had more extensive lesions in the other trunks.

The CASS study (19) produced very significant results, as its registry included 1484 coronary patients with greater than 50% CGRT stenosis randomised to surgery or conservative treatment. The survival rate in the surgical group (1153 patients) was 37% compared with 27% in the non-surgical group (331 patients).

Recently, the 5-year results of the SYNTAX (57) and PRECOMBAT (21) have confirmed the place of bypass surgery in the presence of involvement of the TCCG, in terms of survival and the occurrence of MACCE. This benefit is clearly demonstrated in the presence of a SYNTAX score > 23 and remains at least equivalent below this score. Revascularisation by bypass was more complete and, above all, more durable, compared with the angioplasty group.

Coronary artery bypass grafting is the first-line treatment for unprotected stenoses of the TCCG, because while the anatomical difficulties and severity of the lesions determine the immediate success and long-term results of angioplasty, surgery avoids these difficulties.

Several studies devoted to trunk angioplasty have provided convincing evidence to seriously compete with surgical revascularisation.

Coronary dilatation got off to a difficult start, with severe and discouraging complications (elastic return and dissection during balloon dilatation). The development of stents subsequently reduced these difficulties, but did not solve the problem of restenosis and the high rates of reintervention.

The indications for TCCG angioplasty were therefore limited to protected lesions and patients at very high surgical risk or with limited life expectancy.

The advent of active stents, with their spectacular reduction in restenosis, has led to their being tested in TCCG stenoses.

At the same time as progress has been made in interventional cardiology, surgical revascularisation techniques have also improved, with the development of less invasive techniques, "no-touch aortic" techniques, beating heart surgery, complete arterial revascularisation and improvements in the quality of post-operative resuscitation.

However, in early studies comparing surgery and angioplasty, the advantage of surgery was underestimated because :

- The majority of patients included in these studies were low-risk.

- Few, if any, patients had an all-arterial bypass.

- The inclusion criteria were often "intention to treat". In fact, a large number of patients initially treated with stenting were subsequently bypassed and considered as being treated with angioplasty for the statistical analysis.

The SYNTAX (20) study was designed to compare these two techniques in tri-truncular patients or patients with stenosis of the TCCG.

But even in this large study, surgical revascularisation techniques were not standardised and are far from optimal, whereas in the angioplasty arm of the TCCG, techniques were more homogeneous.

Table VII summarises the mean SYNTAX scores for coronary lesions in the bypass and angioplasty groups in the various studies analysed:

Table VII: SYNTAX SCORE values in the different studies for patients who underwent surgery or angioplasty.

	Average SYNTAX score for the bypass group	Average SYNTAX score for the angioplasty group
Zheng (91)	33.3 +/- 7.8	23.6 +/- 6.7
Patrick (87)	32,7+/-12,9	31,3+/-12,5
Syntax (20)	28,1 ± 12,4	26,7 ± 11,5
Boudriot (22)	23 (14,8-28)	24 (19-29)
Buszman (LE MANS) (56)	25,2± 8,7	24,7± 6,8

Comparative analysis of the two groups at the level of each study analysed showed no significant difference in the mean SYNTAX score between the two groups, given the prospective and randomised nature of these studies.

After an angiographic analysis of the patient's coronary status and lesions, an assessment of the operative risk is essential for the therapeutic decision.

Recent studies have concluded that mortality was similar between angioplasty and surgery, but the occurrence of post-operative stroke was greater in the surgical group, and the risk of intra-stent restenosis and repeat revascularisation were greater in the angioplasty group. Angioplasty therefore appears to have good indications when lesions are limited in number and complexity. It is also a valid alternative when there are significant comorbidities making bypass surgery too risky. (127).

The one-year follow-up of all the series showed that revascularisation of patients with a significant lesion of the TCCG by angioplasty resulted in fewer deaths, MI and strokes than revascularisation by bypass. However, this

difference did not reach the significance threshold except for stroke in the SYNTAX (20).

However, percutaneous revascularisation was responsible for more MACE and repeat revascularisations. Indeed, for major events and apart from the SYNTAX study which found almost the same rate in both groups, all the other studies analysed found a higher rate in the angioplasty group (128) (129) (130). This difference was statistically significant in the LE MANS study population (56).

A study published by Fortuna et al (12) demonstrated the advantage of CABG in reducing 5-year mortality compared with TCA, especially in patients with stenosis of the TCCG and who had bi-truncular or tri-truncular status.

Re-reading the SYNTAX study by integrating both the SYNTAX score and the EuroSCORE provides valuable assistance for therapeutic decisions (131) :

Sinning (132) proposed combining SYNTAX score data with EuroSCORE clinical data and determined 3 levels of risk with a cut-off value:

- EuroSCORE at 7.5% and SYNTAX score at 25: low risk

- EuroSCORE < 7.5% and SYNTAX score < 25: 89.7% MACCE-free survival at 1 year: an intermediate risk.

- A EuroSCORE > 7.5% or SYNTAXscore > 25 to 72.9%: a high risk.

- Euro SCORE > 7.5% and SYNTAX score > 25: MACE-free survival of 47.4%.

Sinning (132) also found a significant difference according to these 3 levels of risk for the following elements taken independently: mortality, need for revascularisation and infarction.

Serruys (20) suggests correlating additive EuroSCORE data with SYNTAX score data to obtain an approach to overall risk. EuroSCORE data have a prognostic value in cardiac surgery but also in angioplasty (133). It identifies 3 levels of risk among patients in the SYNTAX study: low-risk patients: SYNTAX < 33 and EuroSCORE < 6, comparing surgery and angioplasty in patients with common trunk involvement (n = 701), surgery has a higher 3-year mortality than angioplasty (7.5% versus 1.2%, p = 0.0054). For intermediate risk patients: SYNTAX score < 33 and EuroSCORE score > 6 or EuroSCORE score < 6 and SYNTAX score > 33 and for high risk patients SYNTAX score > 33 and EuroSCORE score > 6, there is a benefit to surgery.

Serruys (20) proposes the following algorithm: calculation of the additive EuroSCORE, if it is > 6: surgery, otherwise calculation of the SYNTAX score. If SYNTAX < 22: surgery or angioplasty, between 23-32 if tri-truncular patient: surgery, if isolated common trunk: angioplasty or surgery, for SYNTAX score > 33: surgery.

However, coronary artery bypass grafting had several advantages over angioplasty during a follow-up of 5 to 10 years. The mortality rate was similar between the two groups, but the occurrence of MACE and secondary revascularisation were greater in patients who had undergone angioplasty, hence the superiority of surgery. (49) (106) (125) (134)

Other studies have shown that mortality and the occurrence of MI or stroke are comparable between the two groups, but the advantage of surgery is that the incidence of iterative revascularisation is lower than that observed in the group that received TCA (135) (31) (58).

Table VIII details the results of the various studies that benefited from either a CAP or a TCA.

Table VIII: Different studies comparing surgery and angioplasty.

series	Follow-up (years)	Surgery vs angioplasty
MAIN COMPARE 2008, 2010 (31) (49)	5	Same rate of mortality, coronary events and ischaemic stroke, higher rate of revascularisation with the ATC group.
LE MANS, 2008, 2016 (136) (137)	10	A comparable rate of mortality, myocardial infarction, stroke and repeat revascularisation. Improvement in ejection fraction at 10 years.
SYNTAX, 2010, 2014 (117) (125)	5	A comparable rate of mortality, myocardial infarction, stroke and repeat revascularisation in one year and 5 years.
Boudriot et al, 2011(22)	1	This study favours surgery of the left coronary trunk in 1 year.
PRECOMBAT, 2011, 2015 (21) (138)	5	Higher mortality, myocardial infarction and MACE rates in the ATC group and higher rate of repeat revascularisation.
DELTA, 2012 (50)	3,5	Comparable rates of mortality, myocardial infarction and stroke and high rates of repeat revascularisation with the ATC group

New studies such as PRECOMBAT-2 (139) have studied 2ème generation active stents and compared their impact on morbidity and mortality compared with long-term surgery.

VIII- Indications:

For several years, coronary bypass surgery was considered the gold standard for the treatment of CKGR stenoses, on the basis of the CASS (19).

In the new recommendations, the ATC for ostial and intermediate lesions are class IIa, whereas distal lesions are class IIb, but surgery remains the gold standard in lesions of the left coronary trunk Class I (140, 141).

The SYNTAX study analysed 705 patients with a distal lesion of the TCCG, who were randomised into two subgroups: one group treated surgically with coronary bypass surgery, and the other with TCA. The rate of MACE at 1 year was comparable between the groups (13.7% for the bypass group versus 15.8% for the angioplasty group with $p = 0.44$). (117).

After a follow-up of 5 years, the mortality rate (14.6% for the bypass group versus 12.8% for the angioplasty group with $p = 0.53$) and the rate of MI (4.8% for the bypass group versus 8.2% for the angioplasty group with $p = 0.10$) were not significantly different between the 2 groups. However, the coronary bypass group had a significantly higher rate of stroke than the angioplasty group (4.3% versus 1.5% with $p = 0.03$).

In the case of TCCG involvement with a Syntax score <= 22, there is much more benefit than risk for both treatment strategies, i.e. whatever angioplasty or surgery is chosen.

For patients with a SYNTAX score between 23 and 32, the surgery is class I and the ATC is class IIa.

For patients with a SYNTAX score > 32, coronary bypass surgery was associated with a significant reduction in the use of redux revascularisation (11.6% versus 34.1% with $p < 0.001$).

A meta-analysis (142) evaluated the results at 1 year of 1611 patients divided into 2 groups. There was no significant difference in the mortality rate (4.1% for the coronary bypass group versus 3% for the angioplasty group with p = 0.29), and in the rate of MI (2.8% for the bypass group versus 2.9% for the angioplasty group with p = 0.95), and a higher rate of stroke in the bypass group (1.7% versus 0.1% with p = 0.01).

In a registry of 810 patients with stenosis of the TCCG treated by surgery (335 patients) or by ATC (475 patients), there was no significant difference between the 2 therapeutic options in terms of mortality, MI and stroke after 2 years of follow-up, whereas the risk of re-intervention was significantly lower for the coronary bypass group. (48).

One of the great merits of the SYNTAX (20) study has been to determine an angiographic score which can be used to stratify the interventional risk of each patient.

The SYNTAX score includes several components, such as the number and location of lesions (left common trunk, bifurcation, chronic occlusion, tri-truncular lesions), and their characteristics (tortuosity, calcification, thrombus). This score is useful for making therapeutic decisions, since its severity can determine the prognosis. For surgeons, this SYNTAX score does not affect the prognosis of myocardial revascularisation (coronary artery bypass grafting bypasses coronary lesions regardless of anatomical complexity), but it is very useful for interventional cardiologists.

It is interesting to note that the SYNTAX (20) study found an identical rate of major cardiac events at 3 years between surgery and active stenting when this score was less than or equal to 22.

When it is between 23 and 32, the rate of major cardiac events is identical in the two sub-groups.

Finally, when the SYNTAX score is greater than 33, the advantage goes to surgery.

The "European Coronary Surgery Study" demonstrated, in 59 patients, a 56% reduction in mortality over 5 years as a result of surgery (143).

The mean survival time in the surgical group was 13.3 years, whereas in the other group it was only 6.6 years (19).

A recent randomised clinical trial showed that angioplasty can be an alternative to surgery in patients with favourable anatomical conditions and a high clinical risk. However, this trial demonstrated the advantage of coronary bypass surgery in reducing the incidence of cerebrovascular events (7) (50).

A study published in JACC by Cavalcante et al (84) looked at mortality and the occurrence of MACE at 5 years. For the group of patients with a SYNTAX score between 0 and 32, the occurrence of MACE was similar for the PAC and ATC groups but mortality was significantly higher for the PAC group (p = 0.07), for patients with a SYNTAX score >= 33, the occurrence of MACE was significantly higher for the ATC group (p = 0.007) but mortality was similar for both groups. (26).

The Capodanno study (48) was along the same lines. Analysing data from 819 patients, this author found an identical 2-year mortality rate between the 2 groups when the SYNTAX score was less than or equal to 34, whereas the results were very clearly in favour of surgery (8.5% versus 32.7%) when it was greater than 34.

It is also worth remembering that the recommendations of the European Society of Cardiology (144) on myocardial revascularisation confirm the importance of this score, since they authorise angioplasty with a sufficient level of proof when this score is < 22, whether or not there is a lesion of the TCCG isolated or associated with other coronary lesions.

Over time, however, it became increasingly clear that the SYNTAX score alone was insufficient for clinical decision-making. Other factors such as age, diabetes and renal function can also increase a patient's risk, and these data are not taken into account if we focus solely on the anatomy of the lesions. This is what prompted the development of a new approach, the SYNTAX II score, which takes into account a total of 8 parameters: age, sex, creatinine clearance, left ventricular function, the existence of tri-truncular lesions, involvement of the circumflex, the existence of COPD, and peripheral vascular involvement (145) (82).

Some authors have suggested correlating SYNTAX score data with the most discriminating clinical data: age, creatinine, left ventricular ejection fraction, as demonstrated by Ranucci (146) to determine a Clinical Syntax Score (CSS) (147).

The SYNTAX clinical score has been established to predict the risk of cardiovascular and cerebrovascular events after angioplasty.

Garg (148) evaluated this CSS with encouraging results on 516 patients in the ARTS-II study, determining 3 tertiles of CSS. CSS LOW < 15.6, CSS MID between 15.6 and 27.5 and CSSHIGH > 27.5. At 1 year, 18.7% of patients in the HIGH-risk group had MACE, compared with 7.6% in the MID group and 6.5% in the LOW group, i.e. significantly higher in the high-risk group than in the other two groups.

In addition, the role of the multi-disciplinary approach known as the "Heart Team" must be at the centre of the decision-making process for the treatment of complex coronary lesions, in particular GTCT. (149) (7).

The patient must be at the centre of a discussion between cardiologists, interventional cardiologists, cardiac surgeons and intensive care anaesthetists. The aim is to work together to find the best therapeutic strategy for the patient.

Carlos et al (150) published a prospective study designed to assess the correspondence between the Heart Team decision and the results of the SYNTAX score and SYNTAX score II in tri-truncular patients. Patients recommended for surgery had a higher SYNTAX score (p=0.03) and a significantly higher predicted 4-year mortality in the event of TCA (p=0.04).

IX- Conclusion :

Stenosis of the TCCG is the most serious coronary lesion because of the size of the vascularised myocardial territory and the risk of sudden death that its occlusion can entail.

Atheromatous disease is the main cause of CGRT pathology, and the clinical picture is often noisy.

The seriousness of this condition means that it must be treated rapidly.

Since the 1970s, and more specifically with the results of the CASS (3)the superiority of CABG over medical treatment in the management of TCCG lesions was no longer in doubt. At that time, angioplasty, which was in its infancy, came up against the anatomical complexity of this particular location. The first attempts at percutaneous revascularisation were disappointing. The severity of the lesions was easily circumvented by coronary artery bypass grafting, which became the gold standard treatment for CGRT involvement.

However, the progress made in interventional cardiology since the advent of active stents, the emergence of powerful anti-platelet protocols and the growing experience of operators have enabled interventional cardiologists to take up the challenge of percutaneous revascularisation of TCCG once again.

We are currently witnessing considerable growth in angioplasty of the TCCG worldwide and in our country, in connection with the development and standardisation of angioplasty techniques, the advent of new generations of active stents, and the development of anti-platelet aggregation therapy.

Lastly, a multi-disciplinary approach must be at the heart of the decision-making process for the treatment of complex coronary lesions in GCCT, with the aim of developing a revascularisation strategy targeted at the patient, and which must be the focus of a discussion between cardiologists, interventional cardiologists, cardiac surgeons and anaesthetists.

This 'heart team' approach should be based on risk scores, which are a valuable aid to therapeutic decision-making.

Angiographic scores: SYNTAX score, SYNTAX score II, and SYNTAX clinical score are very useful, particularly if they are combined with a clinical score such as EuroSCORE II, making it possible to select patients much more accurately and guide them towards the most appropriate revascularisation strategy.

Angioplasty with an active stent is an acceptable alternative for patients with isolated involvement of the TCCG and a low SYNTAX score. However, surgery remains the gold standard for revascularisation in patients with tri-truncular disease or TCCG involvement. The patient's opinion also remains essential and must be taken into account to guarantee truly informed and fair consent.

Studies, particularly prospective ones, will enable us to study CGRT stenosis more closely, refine the indications and guide the treatment decision in line with current recommendations.

Bibliography:

1.   DeMots H, Rösch J, McAnulty JH, Rahimtoola SH. Left main coronary artery disease. Cardiovasc Clin. 1977;8(2):201-11.

2.   O'Keefe JH, Hartzler GO, Rutherford BD, McConahay DR, Johnson WL, Giorgi LV, et al. Left main coronary angioplasty: early and late results of 127 acute and elective procedures. Am J Cardiol. 1989 Jul 15;64(3):144-7.

3.   Myers WO, Blackstone EH, Davis K, Foster ED, Kaiser GC. CASS Registry long term surgical survival. Coronary Artery Surgery Study. J Am Coll Cardiol. 1999 Feb;33(2):488-98.

4.   Sangwoo Park, Seung-Jung Park, Duk-Woo Park. Percutaneous Coronary Intervention for Left Main Coronary Artery Disease. Present Status and Future Perspectives. JACC: ASIA, 2022 (2) :119- 138.

5.   Saffioti S, Burzotta F, Coluccia V, Trani C, Bruno P, Massetti M, et al. Usefulness of EuroSCORE systems for risk stratification. J Cardiovasc Med Hagerstown Md. 2015 Feb;16(2):90-9.

6.   Ronnie Ramadan, William E. Boden, Scott Kinlay. Management of Left Main Coronary Artery Disease. Journal of the American Heart Association 2018;7:e008151.

7.   Zheng Z, Xu B, Zhang H, Guan C, Xian Y, Zhao Y, et al. Coronary Artery Bypass Graft Surgery and Percutaneous Coronary Interventions in Patients With Unprotected Left Main Coronary Artery Disease. JACC Cardiovasc Interv. 2016 Jun 13;9(11):1102-11.

8.   Fajadet J, Chieffo A. Current management of left main coronary artery disease. Eur Heart J. 2012 Jan;33(1):36-50b.

9.   Holm F, Lubanda JC, Semrad M, Rohac J, Vondracek V, Miler I, et al. Clinical and operative factors associated with in-hospital mortality after surgery for left coronary artery common trunk stenosis. /data/revues/03980499/00290002/89/ [Internet]. 2008 Mar 20 [cited 2016 Oct 2]; Available from: http://www.em-consulte.com/en/article/125044

10.   Yamanaka O, Hobbs RE. Solitary ostial coronary artery stenosis. Jpn Circ J. 1993 May;57(5):404-10.

11.   Topaz O, Warner M, Lanter P, Soffer A, Burns C, DiSciascio G, et al. Isolated significant left main coronary artery stenosis: angiographic, hemodynamic, and clinical findings in 16 patients. Am Heart J. 1991 Nov;122(5):1308-14.

12.   Fortuna D, Nicolini F, Guastaroba P, De Palma R, Di Bartolomeo S, Saia F, et al. Coronary artery bypass grafting vs percutaneous coronary intervention in a "real-world" setting: a comparative effectiveness study based on propensity score-matched cohorts. Eur J Cardio-Thorac Surg Off J Eur Assoc Cardio-Thorac Surg. 2013 Jul;44(1):e16-24.

13.   Jönsson A, Hammar N, Liska J, Nordqvist T, Ivert T. High mortality after coronary bypass surgery in patients with high-grade left main coronary artery stenosis. Scand Cardiovasc J SCJ. 2006 Jun;40(3):179-85.

14.   Naganuma T, Chieffo A, Meliga E, Capodanno D, Park S-J, Onuma Y, et al. Long-term clinical outcomes after percutaneous coronary intervention versus coronary artery bypass grafting for ostial/midshaft lesions in unprotected left main coronary artery from the DELTA registry: a multicenter registry evaluating percutaneous coronary intervention versus coronary artery bypass grafting for left main treatment. JACC Cardiovasc Interv. 2014 Apr;7(4):354-61.

15.   Fukui T, Takanashi S. Acute Coronary Syndrome Does Not Have a Negative Impact on Outcomes after Coronary Artery Bypass Grafting in Patients with Left Main Disease. Ann Thorac Cardiovasc Surg Off J Assoc Thorac Cardiovasc Surg Asia. 2015;21(3):261-7.

16.   d'Allonnes FR, Corbineau H, Le Breton H, Leclercq C, Leguerrier A, Daubert C. Isolated left main coronary artery stenosis: long term follow up in 106 patients after surgery. Heart Br Card Soc. 2002 Jun;87(6):544-8.

17.   Yu X, He J, Luo Y, Yuan F, Song X, Gao Y, et al. Influence of diabetes mellitus on long-term outcomes of patients with unprotected left main coronary artery disease treated with either drug-eluting stents or coronary artery bypass grafting. Int Heart J. 2015;56(1):43-8.

18.	von Birgelen C, Hartmann M, Mintz GS, Baumgart D, Schmermund A, Erbel R. Relation between progression and regression of atherosclerotic left main coronary artery disease and serum cholesterol levels as assessed with serial long-term (> or =12 months) follow-up intravascular ultrasound. Circulation. 2003 Dec 2;108(22):2757-62.

19.	Caracciolo EA, Davis KB, Sopko G, Kaiser GC, Corley SD, Schaff H, et al. Comparison of surgical and medical group survival in patients with left main equivalent coronary artery disease. Long-term CASS experience. Circulation. 1995 May 1;91(9):2335-44.

20.	Serruys PW, Farooq V, Vranckx P, Girasis C, Brugaletta S, Garcia-Garcia HM, et al. A global risk approach to identify patients with left main or 3-vessel disease who could safely and efficaciously be treated with percutaneous coronary intervention: the SYNTAX Trial at 3 years. JACC Cardiovasc Interv. 2012 Jun;5(6):606-17.

21.	Park S-J, Kim Y-H, Park D-W, Yun S-C, Ahn J-M, Song HG, et al. Randomized trial of stents versus bypass surgery for left main coronary artery disease. N Engl J Med. 2011 May 5;364(18):1718-27.

22.	Boudriot E, Thiele H, Walther T, Liebetrau C, Boeckstegers P, Pohl T, et al. Randomized comparison of percutaneous coronary intervention with sirolimus-eluting stents versus coronary artery bypass grafting in unprotected left main stem stenosis. J Am Coll Cardiol. 2011 Feb 1;57(5):538-45.

23.	Cheng C-I, Lee F-Y, Chang J-P, Hsueh S-K, Hsieh Y-K, Fang C-Y, et al. Long-term outcomes of intervention for unprotected left main coronary artery stenosis: coronary stenting vs coronary artery bypass grafting. Circ J Off J Jpn Circ Soc. 2009 Apr;73(4):705-12.

24.	d'Allonnes FR, Corbineau H, Le Breton H, Leclercq C, Leguerrier A, Daubert C. Isolated left main coronary artery stenosis: long term follow up in 106 patients after surgery. Heart Br Card Soc. 2002 Jun;87(6):544-8.

25.	Seung KB, Park D-W, Kim Y-H, Lee S-W, Lee CW, Hong M-K, et al. Stents versus coronary-artery bypass grafting for left main coronary artery disease. N Engl J Med. 2008 Apr 24;358(17):1781-92.

26.	Cavalcante R, Sotomi Y, Lee CW, Ahn J M, Farooq V, Tateishi H, et al. Outcomes After Percutaneous Coronary Intervention or Bypass Surgery in Patients With Unprotected Left Main Disease. J Am Coll Cardiol. 2016 Sep 6;68(10):999-1009.

27.	el Fawal MA, Berg GA, Wheatley DJ, Harland WA. Sudden coronary death in Glasgow: the severity and distribution of chronic coronary atherosclerotic stenoses. Br Heart J. 1987 May;57(5):420-6.

28.   Seung KB, Park D-W, Kim Y-H, Lee S-W, Lee CW, Hong M-K, et al. Stents versus coronary-artery bypass grafting for left main coronary artery disease. N Engl J Med. 2008 Apr 24;358(17):1781-92.

29.   Lee J-Y, Park D-W, Kim Y-H, Yun S-C, Kim W-J, Kang S-J, et al. Incidence, predictors, treatment, and long-term prognosis of patients with restenosis after drug-eluting stent implantation for unprotected left main coronary artery disease. J Am Coll Cardiol. 2011 Mar 22;57(12):1349-58.

30.   Steg PG, Goldberg RJ, Gore JM, Fox KAA, Eagle KA, Flather MD, et al. Baseline characteristics, management practices, and in-hospital outcomes of patients hospitalized with acute coronary syndromes in the Global Registry of Acute Coronary Events (GRACE). Am J Cardiol. 2002 Aug 15;90(4):358-63.

31.   Seung KB, Park D-W, Kim Y-H, Lee S-W, Lee CW, Hong M-K, et al. Stents versus coronary-artery bypass grafting for left main coronary artery disease. N Engl J Med. 2008 Apr 24;358(17):1781-92.

32.   Carrie D, Derbel F, Delay M, Calazel J, Bernadet P. [Clinical, angiographic aspects and 18-month follow-up of 134 cases of left coronary trunk stenosis]. Arch Mal Coeur Vaiss. 1989 Dec;82(12):2027-33.

33.   Diderholm E, Andrén B, Frostfeldt G, Genberg M, Jernberg T, Lagerqvist B, et al. ST depression in ECG at entry indicates severe coronary lesions and large benefits of an early invasive treatment strategy in unstable coronary artery disease; the FRISC II ECG substudy. The Fast Revascularisation during InStability in Coronary artery disease. Eur Heart J. 2002 Jan;23(1):41-9.

34.   Yamaji H, Iwasaki K, Kusachi S, Murakami T, Hirami R, Hamamoto H, et al. Prediction of acute left main coronary artery obstruction by 12-lead electrocardiography. ST segment elevation in lead aVR with less ST segment elevation in lead V(1). J Am Coll Cardiol. 2001 Nov 1;38(5):1348-54.

35.   Sclarovsky S, Nikus KC, Birnbaum Y, Kjell N. Manifestation of left main coronary artery stenosis is diffuse ST depression in inferior and precordial leads on ECG. J Am Coll Cardiol. 2002 Aug 7;40(3):575-576-577.

36.   Shaw LJ, Peterson ED, Shaw LK, Kesler KL, DeLong ER, Harrell FE, et al. Use of a prognostic treadmill score in identifying diagnostic coronary disease subgroups. Circulation. 1998 Oct 20;98(16):1622-30.

37.   Lanza GA, Mustilli M, Sestito A, Infusino F, Sgueglia GA, Crea F. Diagnostic and prognostic value of ST segment depression limited

to the recovery phase of exercise stress test. Heart Br Card Soc. 2004 Dec;90(12):1417-21.

38. Chikamori T, Doi YL, Yonezawa Y, Yamada M, Seo H, Ozawa T. Noninvasive identification of significant narrowing of the left main coronary artery by dipyridamole thallium scintigraphy. Am J Cardiol. 1991 Aug 15;68(5):472-7.

39. Cohen-Solal A, Leroy G, Paycha F, Haiat R, Juliard JM, Soussana C, et al [Negativity of the exercise thallium test despite tight stenosis of the common trunk of the left coronary artery]. Ann Cardiol Angeiol (Paris). 1992 Apr;41(4):211-3.

40. Ruzsa Z, Pálinkás A, Forster T, Ungi I, Varga A. Angiographically borderline left main coronary artery lesions: correlation of transthoracic doppler echocardiography and intravascular ultrasound: a pilot study. Cardiovasc Ultrasound. 2011;9:19.

41. Caiati C, Zedda N, Cadeddu M, Chen L, Montaldo C, Iliceto S, et al. Detection, location, and severity assessment of left anterior descending coronary artery stenoses by means of contrast-enhanced transthoracic harmonic echo Doppler. Eur Heart J. 2009 Jul;30(14):1797-806.

42. Reichert SL, Visser CA, Koolen JJ, Chapman JV, Angelsen BA, Meyne NG, et al. Transesophageal examination of the left coronary artery with a 7.5 MHz annular array two-dimensional color flow Doppler transducer. J Am Soc Echocardiogr Off Publ Am Soc Echocardiogr. 1990 Apr;3(2):118-24.

43. Flohr T, Bruder H, Stierstorfer K, Simon J, Schaller S, Ohnesorge B. New technical developments in multislice CT, part 2: sub-millimeter 16-slice scanning and increased gantry rotation speed for cardiac imaging. RöFo Fortschritte Auf Dem Geb Röntgenstrahlen Nukl. 2002 Aug;174(8):1022-7.

44. Ferencik M, Moselewski F, Ropers D, Hoffmann U, Baum U, Anders K, et al. Quantitative parameters of image quality in multidetector spiral computed tomographic coronary imaging with submillimeter collimation. Am J Cardiol. 2003 Dec 1;92(11):1257-62.

45. Leschka S, Alkadhi H, Plass A, Desbiolles L, Grünenfelder J, Marincek B, et al. Accuracy of MSCT coronary angiography with 64-slice technology: first experience. Eur Heart J. 2005 Aug;26(15):1482-7.

46. Juwana YB, Wirianta J, Suryapranata H, de Boer M-J. Left main coronary artery stenosis undetected by 64-slice computed

tomography: a word of caution. Neth Heart J Mon J Neth Soc Cardiol Neth Heart Found. 2007;15(7-8):255-6.

47.   El-Menyar AA, Al Suwaidi J, Holmes DR. Left main coronary artery stenosis: state-of-the-art. Curr Probl Cardiol. 2007 Mar;32(3):103-93.

48.   Capodanno D, Di Salvo ME, Cincotta G, Miano M, Tamburino C. Usefulness of the SYNTAX score for predicting clinical outcome after percutaneous coronary intervention of unprotected left main coronary artery disease. Circ Cardiovasc Interv. 2009 Aug;2(4):302-8.

49.   Park D-W, Seung KB, Kim Y-H, Lee J-Y, Kim W-J, Kang S-J, et al. Long-term safety and efficacy of stenting versus coronary artery bypass grafting for unprotected left main coronary artery disease: 5-year results from the MAIN-COMPARE (Revascularization for Unprotected Left Main Coronary Artery Stenosis: Comparison of Percutaneous Coronary Angioplasty Versus Surgical Revascularization) registry. J Am Coll Cardiol. 2010 Jul 6;56(2):117-24.

50.   Chieffo A, Meliga E, Latib A, Park S-J, Onuma Y, Capranzano P, et al. Drug-eluting stent for left main coronary artery disease. The DELTA registry: a multicenter registry evaluating percutaneous coronary intervention versus coronary artery bypass grafting for left main treatment. JACC Cardiovasc Interv. 2012 Jul;5(7):718-27.

51.   Chieffo A, Magni V, Latib A, Maisano F, Ielasi A, Montorfano M, et al. 5-year outcomes following percutaneous coronary intervention with drug-eluting stent implantation versus coronary artery bypass graft for unprotected left main coronary artery lesions the Milan experience. JACC Cardiovasc Interv. 2010 Jun;3(6):595-601.

52.   Jönsson A, Ivert T, Svane B, Liska J, Jakobsson K, Hammar N. Classification of left main coronary obstruction--feasibility of surgical angioplasty and survival after coronary artery bypass surgery. Cardiovasc Surg Lond Engl. 2003 Dec;11(6):497-505.

53.   Kappetein AP, Dawkins KD, Mohr FW, Morice MC, Mack MJ, Russell ME, et al. Current percutaneous coronary intervention and coronary artery bypass grafting practices for three-vessel and left main coronary artery disease. Insights from the SYNTAX run-in phase. Eur J Cardio-Thorac Surg Off J Eur Assoc Cardio-Thorac Surg. 2006 Apr;29(4):486-91.

54.   Rollé F, Christidès C, Cornu E, Virot P, Doumeix JJ, Cassat C, et al [Significant stenosis of the common trunk of the left coronary artery. Retrospective study of 227 cases]. Arch Mal Coeur Vaiss. 1994 Jul;87(7):899-905.

55.   Carrie D, Derbel F, Delay M, Calazel J, Bernadet P. [Clinical, angiographic aspects and 18-month follow-up of 134 cases of left coronary trunk stenosis]. Arch Mal Coeur Vaiss. 1989 Dec;82(12):2027-33.

56.   Buszman PE, Buszman PP, Kiesz RS, Bochenek A, Trela B, Konkolewska M, et al. Early and long-term results of unprotected left main coronary artery stenting: the LE MANS (Left Main Coronary Artery Stenting) registry. J Am Coll Cardiol. 2009 Oct 13;54(16):1500-11.

57.   Mohr FW, Morice M-C, Kappetein AP, Feldman TE, Ståhle E, Colombo A, et al. Coronary artery bypass graft surgery versus percutaneous coronary intervention in patients with three-vessel disease and left main coronary disease: 5-year follow-up of the randomised, clinical SYNTAX trial. Lancet Lond Engl. 2013 Feb 23;381(9867):629-38.

58.   Serruys PW, Morice M-C, Kappetein AP, Colombo A, Holmes DR, Mack MJ, et al. Percutaneous coronary intervention versus coronary-artery bypass grafting for severe coronary artery disease. N Engl J Med. 2009 Mar 5;360(10):961-72.

59.   Arima M, Kanoh T, Okazaki S, Iwama Y, Matsuda S, Nakazato Y. Long-term clinical and angiographic follow-up in patients with isolated ostial stenosis of the left coronary artery. Circ J Off J Jpn Circ Soc. 2009 Jul;73(7):1271-7.

60.   Trnka KE, Febres-Roman PR, Cadigan RA, Crone RA, Williams TH. Total occlusion of the left main coronary artery: clinical and catheterization findings. Clin Cardiol. 1980 Oct;3(5):352-5.

61.   Kim D, Guthaner DF, Wexler L, Gonzalez-Lavin L. Isolated total occlusion of the left main coronary artery. AJR Am J Roentgenol. 1983 Dec;141(6):1304-6.

62.   Shahian DM, Butterly JR, Malacoff RF. Total obstruction of the left main coronary artery. Ann Thorac Surg. 1988 Sep;46(3):317-20.

63.   Nishimura RA, Higano ST, Holmes DR. Use of intracoronary ultrasound imaging for assessing left main coronary artery disease. Mayo Clin Proc. 1993 Feb;68(2):134-40.

64.   Gil RJ, Gziut AI, Prati F, Witkowski A, Kubica J. Threshold parameters of left main coronary artery stem stenosis based on

intracoronary ultrasound examination. Kardiol Pol. 2005 Sep;63(3):223-231-233.

65.   Bech GJ, Droste H, Pijls NH, De Bruyne B, Bonnier JJ, Michels HR, et al. Value of fractional flow reserve in making decisions about bypass surgery for equivocal left main coronary artery disease. Heart Br Card Soc. 2001 Nov;86(5):547-52.

66.   Zimmern SH, Rogers WJ, Bream PR, Chaitman BR, Bourassa MG, Davis KA, et al. Total occlusion of the left main coronary artery: the Coronary Artery Surgery Study (CASS) experience. Am J Cardiol. 1982 Jun;49(8):2003-10.

67.   Yusuf S, Zucker D, Peduzzi P, Fisher LD, Takaro T, Kennedy JW, et al. Effect of coronary artery bypass graft surgery on survival: overview of 10-year results from randomised trials by the Coronary Artery Bypass Graft Surgery Trialists Collaboration. Lancet Lond Engl. 1994 Aug 27;344(8922):563-70.

68.   Yu X, He J, Luo Y, Yuan F, Song X, Gao Y, et al. Influence of diabetes mellitus on long-term outcomes of patients with unprotected left main coronary artery disease treated with either drug-eluting stents or coronary artery bypass grafting. Int Heart J. 2015;56(1):43-8.

69.   Maziak DE, Rao V, Christakis GT, Buth KJ, Sever J, Fremes SE, et al. Can patients with left main stenosis wait for coronary artery bypass grafting? Ann Thorac Surg. 1996 Feb;61(2):552-7.

70.   da Rocha ASC, da Silva PRD. Can patients with left main coronary artery disease wait for myocardial revascularization surgery? Arq Bras Cardiol. 2003 Feb;80(2):191-3, 187-90.

71.   Murzi M, Caputo M, Aresu G, Duggan S, Miceli A, Glauber M, et al. On-pump and off-pump coronary artery bypass grafting in patients with left main stem disease: a propensity score analysis. J Thorac Cardiovasc Surg. 2012 Jun;143(6):1382-8.

72.   Carpentier A, Loulmet D, Aupecle B, Berrebi A, Relland J. Computer-assisted cardiac surgery. Lancet Lond Engl. 1999 Jan 30;353(9150):379-80.

73.   Falk V, Diegeler A, Walther T, Banusch J, Brucerius J, Raumans J, et al. Total endoscopic computer enhanced coronary artery bypass grafting. Eur J Cardio-Thorac Surg Off J Eur Assoc Cardio-Thorac Surg. 2000 Jan;17(1):38-45.

74.   Effler DB, Sones FM, Favaloro R, Groves LK. Coronary endarterotomy with patch-graft reconstruction: clinical experience with 34 cases. Ann Surg. 1965 Oct;162(4):590-601.

75.   Sabiston DC, Ebert PA, Friesinger GC, Ross RS, Sinclair-Smith B. Proximal endarterectomy, arterial reconstruction for coronary occlusion at aortic origin. Arch Surg Chic Ill 1960. 1965 Nov;91(5):758-64.

76.   Jedaden O, Eker A, Durand De Gevigney G, Rossi R, Montagna P, Ossette J, et al. Plastie chirurgicale des troncs coronaires : une alternative aux techniques de pontages. Arch Mal Coeur Vaiss. 1994;87(10):1325-9.

77.   Martinovic I, Greve H. Surgical reconstruction of the left main coronary artery with patch-angioplasty. J Cardiothorac Surg. 2011;6:24.

78.   Maureira P, Vanhuyse F, Lekehal M, Tran N, Carteaux J-P, Villemot J-P. Left main coronary disease treated by direct surgical angioplasty: long-term results. Ann Thorac Surg. 2010 Apr;89(4):1151-7.

79.   Bernal-Aragón R, Sáenz-Rodríguez R, Orozco-Hernández E, Guzmán-Delgado N, Aragón-Manjarrez R, Hernández-Alvídrez A. [Coronary endarterectomy experience in myocardial revascularization]. Cir Cir. 2015 Aug;83(4):273-8.

80.   Bagheri A, Masoumi A, Bagheri J. Early Outcomes of Coronary Endarterectomy in Patients Undergoing Coronary Artery Bypass Surgery. Heart Surg Forum. 2016;19(2):E059-63.

81.   Beauford RB, Saunders CR, Lunceford TA, Niemeier LA, Shah S, Karanam R, et al. Multivessel off-pump revascularization in patients with significant left main coronary artery stenosis: early and midterm outcome analysis. J Card Surg. 2005 Apr;20(2):112-8.

82.   Yeatman M, Caputo M, Ascione R, Ciulli F, Angelini GD. Off-pump coronary artery bypass surgery for critical left main stem disease: safety, efficacy and outcome. Eur J Cardio-Thorac Surg Off J Eur Assoc Cardio-Thorac Surg. 2001 Mar;19(3):239-44.

83.   Sianos G, Morel M-A, Kappetein AP, Morice M-C, Colombo A, Dawkins K, et al. The SYNTAX Score: an angiographic tool grading the complexity of coronary artery disease. EuroIntervention J Eur Collab Work Group Interv Cardiol Eur Soc Cardiol. 2005 Aug;1(2):219-27.

84.   Liu T, Lu I-K, Gan H-L, Zhang J-Q, Huang F-J, Gu C-X, et al. High volume practice proved the safety of off-pump coronary artery bypass

surgery in left main coronary artery lesions: a two-year single center experience. Chin Med J (Engl). 2012 Nov;125(21):3861-7.

85.   Brener SJ, Lytle BW, Casserly IP, Schneider JP, Topol EJ, Lauer MS. Propensity analysis of long-term survival after surgical or percutaneous revascularization in patients with multivessel coronary artery disease and high-risk features. Circulation. 2004 May 18;109(19):2290-5.

86.   Ait Houssa M, Moutakiallah Y, Abdou A, Selkane C, Amahzoune B, Drissi M, et al. Results of coronary bypass surgery in left ventricular dysfunction (comparison of beating heart and bypass surgery). Ann Cardiol Aneiology. 2013 Aug;62(4):241-7.

87.   Yin Y, Xin X, Geng T, Xu Z. Clinical comparison of percutaneous coronary intervention with domestic drug-eluting stents versus off pump coronary artery bypass grafting in unprotected left main coronary artery disease. Int J Clin Exp Med. 2015;8(8):14376-82.

88.   Borde DP, Asegaonkar B, Apsingekar P, Khade S, Futane S, Khodve B, et al. Intraoperative conversion to on-pump coronary artery bypass grafting is independently associated with higher mortality in patients undergoing off-pump coronary artery bypass grafting: A propensity-matched analysis. Ann Card Anaesth. 2016 Sep;19(3):475-80.

89.   Afrasiabirad A, Safaie N, Montazergaem H. On-pump beating coronary artery bypass in high risk coronary patients. Iran J Med Sci. 2015 Jan;40(1):40-4.

90.   Cohen HA, Zenati M, Smith AJ, Lee JS, Chough S, Jafar Z, et al. Feasibility of combined percutaneous transluminal angioplasty and minimally invasive direct coronary artery bypass in patients with multivessel coronary artery disease. Circulation. 1998 Sep 15;98(11):1048-50.

91.   Rodríguez Hernández JE, López Gude MJ, Rufilanchas Sánchez JJ, Maroto Castellanos LC, González-Trevilla AA, Tascón Pérez J. [Hybrid revascularization]. Rev Esp Cardiol. 1999 Nov;52(11):898-902.

92.   Hu F-B, Cui L-Q. Short-term clinical outcomes after hybrid coronary revascularization versus off-pump coronary artery bypass for the treatment of multivessel or left main coronary artery disease: a meta-analysis. Coron Artery Dis. 2015 Sep;26(6):526-34.

93.   Kvidal P, Bergström R, Hörte LG, Ståhle E. Observed and relative survival after aortic valve replacement. J Am Coll Cardiol. 2000 Mar 1;35(3):747-56.

94.   Gilbert T, Orr W, Banning AP. Surgery for aortic stenosis in severely symptomatic patients older than 80 years: experience in a single UK centre. Heart Br Card Soc. 1999 Aug;82(2):138-42.

95.   Hannan EL, Racz MJ, Jones RH, Gold JP, Ryan TJ, Hafner JP, et al. Predictors of mortality for patients undergoing cardiac valve replacements in New York State. Ann Thorac Surg. 2000 Oct;70(4):1212-8.

96.   Grover FL, Edwards FH. Similarity between the STS and New York State databases for valvular heart disease. Ann Thorac Surg. 2000 Oct;70(4):1143-4.

97.   Iung B, Drissi MF, Michel PL, de Pamphilis O, Tsezana R, Cormier B, et al. Prognosis of valve replacement for aortic stenosis with or without coexisting coronary heart disease: a comparative study. J Heart Valve Dis. 1993 Jul;2(4):430-9.

98.   Jamieson WR, Edwards FH, Schwartz M, Bero JW, Clark RE, Grover FL. Risk stratification for cardiac valve replacement. National Cardiac Surgery Database. Database Committee of The Society of Thoracic Surgeons. Ann Thorac Surg. 1999 Apr;67(4):943-51.

99.   Zembala MO, Filipiak K, Ciesla D, Pacholewicz J, Hrapkowicz T, Knapik P, et al. Surgical treatment of left main disease and severe carotid stenosis: does the off-pump technique provide a better outcome? Eur J Cardio-Thorac Surg Off J Eur Assoc Cardio-Thorac Surg. 2013 Mar;43(3):541-548; discussion 548.

100.   Sher-I-Murtaza M, Baig MAR, Raheel HMA. Early outcome of Coronary Artery Bypass Graft Surgery in patients with significant Left Main Stem stenosis at a tertiary cardiac care center. Pak J Med Sci. 2015 Aug;31(4):909-14.

101.   Brann S, Martineau R, Cartier R. Left main coronary artery stenosis: early experience with surgical revascularization without cardiopulmonary bypass. J Cardiovasc Surg (Torino). 2000 Apr;41(2):175-9.

102.   Burgos JD, Munoz OC, Mukherjee D. Emergency intervention for unprotected left main coronary artery stenosis: case report and review of the literature. Hell J Cardiol HJC Hellēnikē Kardiologikē Epitheōrēsē. 2011 Dec;52(6):545-8.

103.	Lu JCY, Grayson AD, Pullan DM. On-pump versus off-pump surgical revascularization for left main stem stenosis: risk adjusted outcomes. Ann Thorac Surg. 2005 Jul;80(1):136-42.

104.	Brilakis ES, Wright RS, Kopecky SL, Mavrogiorgos NC, Reeder GS, Rihal CS, et al. Association of the PURSUIT risk score with predischarge ejection fraction, angiographic severity of coronary artery disease, and mortality in a nonselected, community-based population with non-ST-elevation acute myocardial infarction. Am Heart J. 2003 Nov;146(5):811-8.

105.	Ellis SG, Hill CM, Lytle BW. Spectrum of surgical risk for left main coronary stenoses: benchmark for potentially competing percutaneous therapies. Am Heart J. 1998 Feb;135(2 Pt 1):335-8.

106.	Comparison of coronary bypass surgery with angioplasty in patients with multivessel disease. The Bypass Angioplasty Revascularization Investigation (BARI) Investigators. N Engl J Med. 1996 Jul 25;335(4):217-25.

107.	Farkouh ME, Domanski M, Sleeper LA, Siami FS, Dangas G, Mack M, et al. Strategies for multivessel revascularization in patients with diabetes. N Engl J Med. 2012 Dec 20;367(25):2375-84.

108.	Sabik JF, Blackstone EH, Firstenberg M, Lytle BW. A benchmark for evaluating innovative treatment of left main coronary disease. Circulation. 2007 Sep 11;116(11 Suppl):I232-239.

109.	Gomberg J, Klein LW, Seelaus P, Parr GV, Agarwal JB, Helfant RH. Surgical revascularization of left main coronary artery stenosis: determinants of perioperative and long-term outcome in the 1980s. Am Heart J. 1988 Aug;116(2 Pt 1):440-6.

110.	Sevray B, Logeais Y, Chaperon J, Leguerrier A, Rioux C, Langanay T, et al [Changes in operative risk and its predictive factors in coronary surgery]. Arch Mal Coeur Vaiss. 1995 Jun;88(6):847-54.

111.	Chaitman BR, Rogers WJ, Davis K, Tyras DH, Berger R, Bourassa MG, et al. Operative risk factors in patients with left main coronary-artery disease. N Engl J Med. 1980 Oct 23;303(17):953-7.

112.	Bouchart F, Tabley A, Litzler PY, Haas-Hubscher C, Bessou JP, Soyer R. Myocardial revascularization in patients with severe ischemic left ventricular dysfunction. Long term follow-up in 141 patients. Eur J

Cardio-Thorac Surg Off J Eur Assoc Cardio-Thorac Surg. 2001 Dec;20(6):1157-62.

113.   Pan Y, Qiu Q, Chen F, Li X, Yu X, Luo Y, et al. Impact of chronic kidney disease on patients with unprotected left main coronary artery disease treated with coronary artery bypass grafting or drug-eluting stents. Coron Artery Dis. 2016 Nov;27(7):535-42.

114   Mangano CM, Diamondstone LS, Ramsay JG, Aggarwal A, Herskowitz A, Mangano DT. Renal dysfunction after myocardial revascularization: risk factors, adverse outcomes, and hospital resource utilization. The Multicenter Study of Perioperative Ischemia Research Group. Ann Intern Med. 1998 Feb 1;128(3):194-203.

115.   Crochet DP, Campeau L, Petitclerc R. [Stenosis of the common trunk of the left coronary artery. Importance of associated coronary involvement. I. Angiographic study]. Coeur Med Interne. 1975 Jun;14(2):199-204.

116.   Rollé F, Christidès C, Cornu E, Virot P, Doumeix JJ, Cassat C, et al [Significant stenosis of the common trunk of the left coronary artery. Retrospective study of 227 cases]. Arch Mal Coeur Vaiss. 1994 Jul;87(7):899-905.

117.   Morice M-C, Serruys PW, Kappetein AP, Feldman TE, Ståhle E, Colombo A, et al. Outcomes in patients with de novo left main disease treated with either percutaneous coronary intervention using paclitaxel-eluting stents or coronary artery bypass graft treatment in the Synergy Between Percutaneous Coronary Intervention with TAXUS and Cardiac Surgery (SYNTAX) trial. Circulation. 2010 Jun 22;121(24):2645-53.

118.   Rexius H, Brandrup-Wognsen G, Nilsson J, Odén A, Jeppsson A. A simple score to assess mortality risk in patients waiting for coronary artery bypass grafting. Ann Thorac Surg. 2006 Feb;81(2):577-82.

119.   Deviri E, Arbell D, Glick Y, Deeb M, Yizhar U, Grunfeld G, et al. Warm blood cardioplegia for patients undergoing revascularization for left main coronary artery disease. Thorac Cardiovasc Surg. 1993 Oct;41(5):280-3.

120   Rollé F, Christidès C, Cornu E, Virot P, Doumeix JJ, Cassat C, et al [Significant stenosis of the common trunk of the left coronary artery. Retrospective study of 227 cases]. Arch Mal Coeur Vaiss. 1994 Jul;87(7):899-905.

121.   Sher-i-Murtaza M, Baig MAR, Raheel HMA. Early outcome of Coronary Artery Bypass Graft Surgery in patients with significant Left Main Stem stenosis at a tertiary cardiac care center. Pak J Med Sci

[Internet]. 1969 Dec 31 [cited 2016 Oct 4];31(4). Available from: http://pjms.com.pk/index.php/pjms/article/view/7597

122.   Ocete G, Guerrero A, Diaz-Peletier R, Burgos J, Bouza E, De Miguel C. Experience in the treatment of osseous hydatidosis. Int Orthop. 1986 Jun;10(2):141-5.

123.   Eagle KA, Guyton RA, Davidoff R, Edwards FH, Ewy GA, Gardner TJ, et al. ACC/AHA 2004 guideline update for coronary artery bypass graft surgery: summary article: a report of the American College of Cardiology/American Heart Association Task Force on Practice Guidelines (Committee to Update the 1999 Guidelines for Coronary Artery Bypass Graft Surgery). Circulation. 2004 Aug 31;110(9):1168-76.

124   Yip HK, Wu CJ, Chen MC, Chang HW, Hsieh KY, Hang CL, et al. Effect of primary angioplasty on total or subtotal left main occlusion: analysis of incidence, clinical features, outcomes, and prognostic determinants. Chest. 2001 Oct;120(4):1212-7.

125   Morice M-C, Serruys PW, Kappetein AP, Feldman TE, Ståhle E, Colombo A, et al. Five-year outcomes in patients with left main disease treated with either percutaneous coronary intervention or coronary artery bypass grafting in the synergy between percutaneous coronary intervention with taxus and cardiac surgery trial. Circulation. 2014 Jun 10;129(23):2388-94.

126.   Berger PB, Velianou JL, Aslanidou Vlachos H, Feit F, Jacobs AK, Faxon DP, et al. Survival following coronary angioplasty versus coronary artery bypass surgery in anatomic subsets in which coronary artery bypass surgery improves survival compared with medical therapy. Results from the Bypass Angioplasty Revascularization Investigation (BARI). J Am Coll Cardiol. 2001 Nov 1;38(5):1440-9.

127.   Lee PH, Ahn J-M, Chang M, Baek S, Yoon S-H, Kang S-J, et al. Left Main Coronary Artery Disease: Secular Trends in Patient Characteristics, Treatments, and Outcomes. J Am Coll Cardiol. 2016 Sep 13;68(11):1233-46.

128.   Lee MS, Kapoor N, Jamal F, Czer L, Aragon J, Forrester J, et al. Comparison of coronary artery bypass surgery with percutaneous coronary intervention with drug-eluting stents for unprotected left main coronary artery disease. J Am Coll Cardiol. 2006 Feb 21;47(4):864-70.

129.   Silvestri M, Barragan P, Sainsous J, Bayet G, Simeoni JB, Roquebert PO, et al. Unprotected left main coronary artery stenting:

immediate and medium-term outcomes of 140 elective procedures. J Am Coll Cardiol. 2000 May;35(6):1543-50.

130. Black A, Cortina R, Bossi I, Choussat R, Fajadet J, Marco J. Unprotected left main coronary artery stenting: correlates of midterm survival and impact of patient selection. J Am Coll Cardiol. 2001 Mar 1;37(3):832-8.

131 Zhao M, Stampf S, Valina C, Kienzle R-P, Ferenc M, Gick M, et al. Role of euroSCORE II in predicting long-term outcome after percutaneous catheter intervention for coronary triple vessel disease or left main stenosis. Int J Cardiol. 2013 Oct 9;168(4):3273-9.

132. Sinning J-M, Stoffel V, Grube E, Nickenig G, Werner N. Combination of angiographic and clinical characteristics for the prediction of clinical outcomes in patients undergoing unprotected left main coronary artery stenting. Clin Res Cardiol Off J Ger Card Soc. 2012 Jun;101(6):477-85.

133. Kim Y-H, Ahn J-M, Park D-W, Lee B-K, Lee CW, Hong M-K, et al. EuroSCORE as a predictor of death and myocardial infarction after unprotected left main coronary stenting. Am J Cardiol. 2006 Dec 15;98(12):1567-70.

134. Park D-W, Kim Y-H, Yun S-C, Lee J-Y, Kim W-J, Kang S-J, et al. Long-term outcomes after stenting versus coronary artery bypass grafting for unprotected left main coronary artery disease: 10-year results of bare-metal stents and 5-year results of drug-eluting stents from the ASAN-MAIN (ASAN Medical Center-Left MAIN Revascularization) Registry. J Am Coll Cardiol. 2010 Oct 19;56(17):1366-75.

135. Chieffo A, Morici N, Maisano F, Bonizzoni E, Cosgrave J, Montorfano M, et al. Percutaneous treatment with drug-eluting stent implantation versus bypass surgery for unprotected left main stenosis: a single-center experience. Circulation. 2006 May 30;113(21):2542-7.

136. Buszman PE, Kiesz SR, Bochenek A, Peszek-Przybyla E, Szkrobka I, Debinski M, et al. Acute and late outcomes of unprotected left main stenting in comparison with surgical revascularization. J Am Coll Cardiol. 2008 Feb 5;51(5):538-45.

137. Buszman PE, Buszman PP, Banasiewicz-Szkróbka I, Milewski KP, Żurakowski A, Orlik B, et al. Left Main Stenting in Comparison With Surgical Revascularization: 10-Year Outcomes of the

(Left Main Coronary Artery Stenting) LE MANS Trial. JACC Cardiovasc Interv. 2016 Feb 22;9(4):318-27.

138.   Ahn J-M, Roh J-H, Kim Y-H, Park D-W, Yun S-C, Lee PH, et al. Randomized Trial of Stents Versus Bypass Surgery for Left Main Coronary Artery Disease: 5-Year Outcomes of the PRECOMBAT Study. J Am Coll Cardiol. 2015 May 26;65(20):2198-206.

139   Kim Y-H, Park D-W, Ahn J-M, Yun S-C, Song HG, Lee J-Y, et al. Everolimus-eluting stent implantation for unprotected left main coronary artery stenosis. The PRECOMBAT-2 (Premier of Randomized Comparison of Bypass Surgery versus Angioplasty Using Sirolimus-Eluting Stent in Patients with Left Main Coronary Artery Disease) study. JACC Cardiovasc Interv. 2012 Jul;5(7):708-17.

140   Authors/Task Force members, Windecker S, Kolh P, Alfonso F, Collet J-P, Cremer J, et al. 2014 ESC/EACTS Guidelines on myocardial revascularization: The Task Force on Myocardial Revascularization of the European Society of Cardiology (ESC) and the European Association for Cardio-Thoracic Surgery (EACTS)Developed with the special contribution of the European Association of Percutaneous Cardiovascular Interventions (EAPCI). Eur Heart J. 2014 Oct 1;35(37):2541-619.

141.   Levine GN, Bates ER, Blankenship JC, Bailey SR, Bittl JA, Cercek B, et al. 2011 ACCF/AHA/SCAI Guideline for Percutaneous Coronary Intervention: executive summary: a report of the American College of Cardiology Foundation/American Heart Association Task Force on Practice Guidelines and the Society for Cardiovascular Angiography and Interventions. Catheter Cardiovasc Interv Off J Soc Card Angiogr Interv. 2012 Feb 15;79(3):453-95.

142.   Capodanno D, Stone GW, Morice MC, Bass TA, Tamburino C. Percutaneous coronary intervention versus coronary artery bypass graft surgery in left main coronary artery disease: a meta-analysis of randomized clinical data. J Am Coll Cardiol. 2011 Sep 27;58(14):1426-32.

143.   Long-term results of prospective randomised study of coronary artery bypass surgery in stable angina pectoris. European Coronary Surgery Study Group. Lancet Lond Engl. 1982 Nov 27;2(8309):1173-80.

144   Task Force on Myocardial Revascularization of the European Society of Cardiology (ESC) and the European Association for Cardio-Thoracic Surgery (EACTS), European Association for Percutaneous Cardiovascular Interventions (EAPCI), Wijns W, Kolh P, Danchin N, Di

Mario C, et al. Guidelines on myocardial revascularization. Eur Heart J. 2010 Oct;31(20):2501-55.

145.   Farooq V, van Klaveren D, Steyerberg EW, Meliga E, Vergouwe Y, Chieffo A, et al. Anatomical and clinical characteristics to guide decision making between coronary artery bypass surgery and percutaneous coronary intervention for individual patients: development and validation of SYNTAX score II. Lancet Lond Engl. 2013 Feb 23;381(9867):639-50.

146.   Ranucci M, Castelvecchio S, Menicanti L, Frigiola A, Pelissero G. Risk of assessing mortality risk in elective cardiac operations: age, creatinine, ejection fraction, and the law of parsimony. Circulation. 2009 Jun 23;119(24):3053-61.

147.   Garg S, Sarno G, Garcia-Garcia HM, Girasis C, Wykrzykowska J, Dawkins KD, et al. A new tool for the risk stratification of patients with complex coronary artery disease: the Clinical SYNTAX Score. Circ Cardiovasc Interv. 2010 Aug;3(4):317-26.

148.   Serruys PW, Ong ATL, Morice M-C, De Bruyne B, Colombo A, Macaya C, et al. Arterial Revascularisation Therapies Study Part II - Sirolimus-eluting stents for the treatment of patients with multivessel de novo coronary artery lesions. EuroIntervention J Eur Collab Work Group Interv Cardiol Eur Soc Cardiol. 2005 Aug;1(2):147-56.

149.   Center for History and New Media. Quick Start Guide [Internet]. Available from: http://zotero.org/support/quick_start_guide.

150   Campos CM, Stanetic BM, Farooq V, Walsh S, Ishibashi Y, Onuma Y, et al. Risk stratification in 3-vessel coronary artery disease: Applying the SYNTAX Score II in the Heart Team Discussion of the SYNTAX II trial. Catheter Cardiovasc Interv Off J Soc Card Angiogr Interv. 2015 Nov 15;86(6): E229-238.

Table of Contents

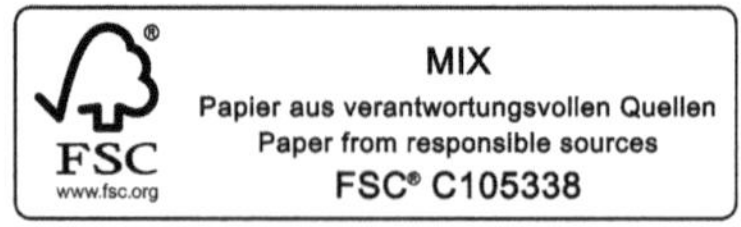

Printed by Books on Demand GmbH, Norderstedt / Germany